FUN SEX

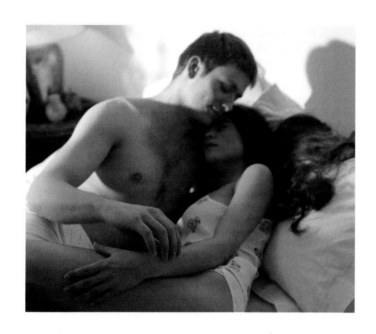

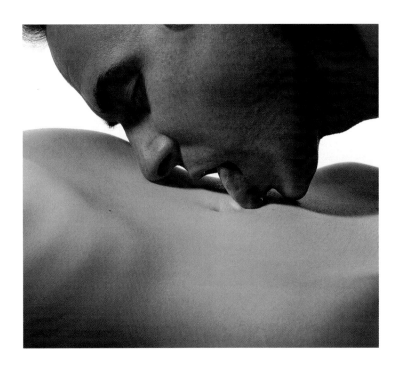

THIS IS A CARLTON BOOK

Text and Design © Carlton Books Limited, 1999
Photography: Alastair Hughes, John Mason, Susanna Price, Alan
Randall/©Carlton Books Ltd.
This edition published by Carlton Books Limited, 1999
A CIP catalogue record for this book is available from the British Library

ISBN 1 85868 831 0

Project Editor: Camilla MacWhannell
Project art direction: Diane Spender
Design and Editorial: Paul Middleton & Warren Lapworth
Production: Alexia Turner
Picture Research: Lorna Ainger

Printed and bound in Italy

FUN SEX

Exciting ideas for better love making

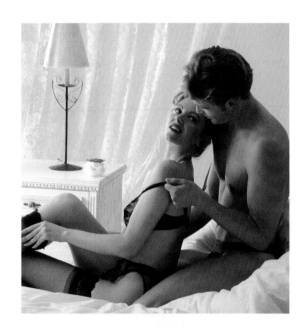

SALLY BISHOP

CARLTON

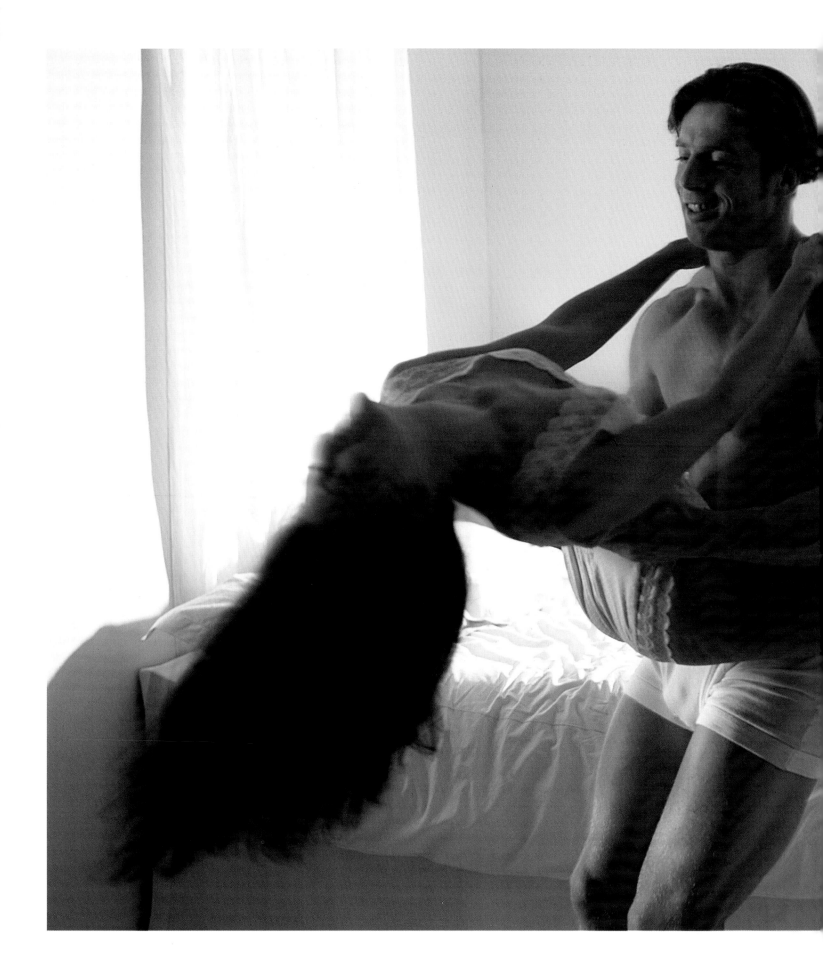

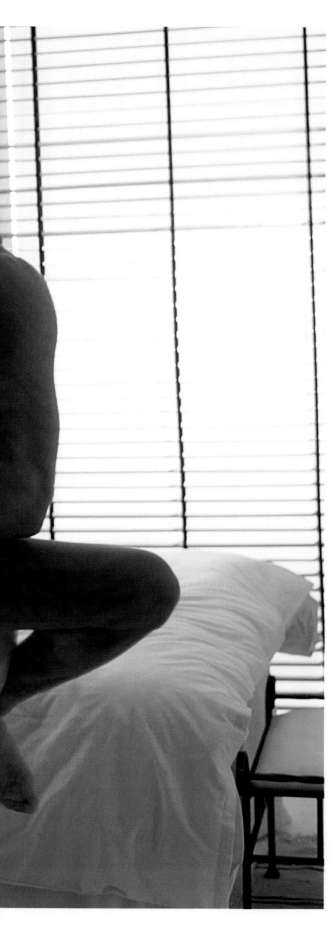

CONTENTS

INTRODUCTION

Humour is a great seducer. How many times have you heard someone say they were 'laughed into bed'? And what this proves is that if you are relaxed about sex, you enjoy it. Likewise, if you enjoy sex, you are relaxed. Sounds too simple? Well, if you're used to everything in life being fast and furious, having deadlines and being deadly serious, you probably take your love-making with a spoonful of gravity, too. Which is an awful shame, because it's the one thing in life you can happily depend on. And the word 'happily' is used for a reason – the bedroom should be a happy place full of happy times.

When it seems that your world has collapsed around you, how can you beat the gorgeous intimacy of being entwined with the one you love? Sadly, a lot of the fun has gone out of people's lives. And that applies to their sex lives, too. We are all so concerned with time-keeping, what others think of us – and indeed, what we think about ourselves – and competition in all fields of modern living that fun gets forgotten. Yet sex is the best and most natural fun you can have.

Which is why this book has been written. It is titled Fun Sex, and here's why: Because it makes sex FUN again. We have had far too many sex manuals, too many worthy volumes that explore the hidden depths of sexuality and plunge into the psychology of it all. They are all so serious. Previous works have often been laughable – but for all the wrong reasons.

This book is different. We should indeed laugh and joke about sex, and talk openly about it. Perhaps the way to treat sex is in a serious fun way. This book tries to avoid sexual psycho-babble and uses words and terms we can all understand. Hopefully, the lighthearted vein doesn't detract from the meaningfulness of a good, honest sexual relationship, but enhances it.

So as you flip through the pages on Fantasies, Fabulous Feelings and Fulfilment, find some fancy ideas to colour your love life.

Above all, have Fun Sex.

RIGHT: Making love with the one you love is natural, normal and utterly life-enhancing.

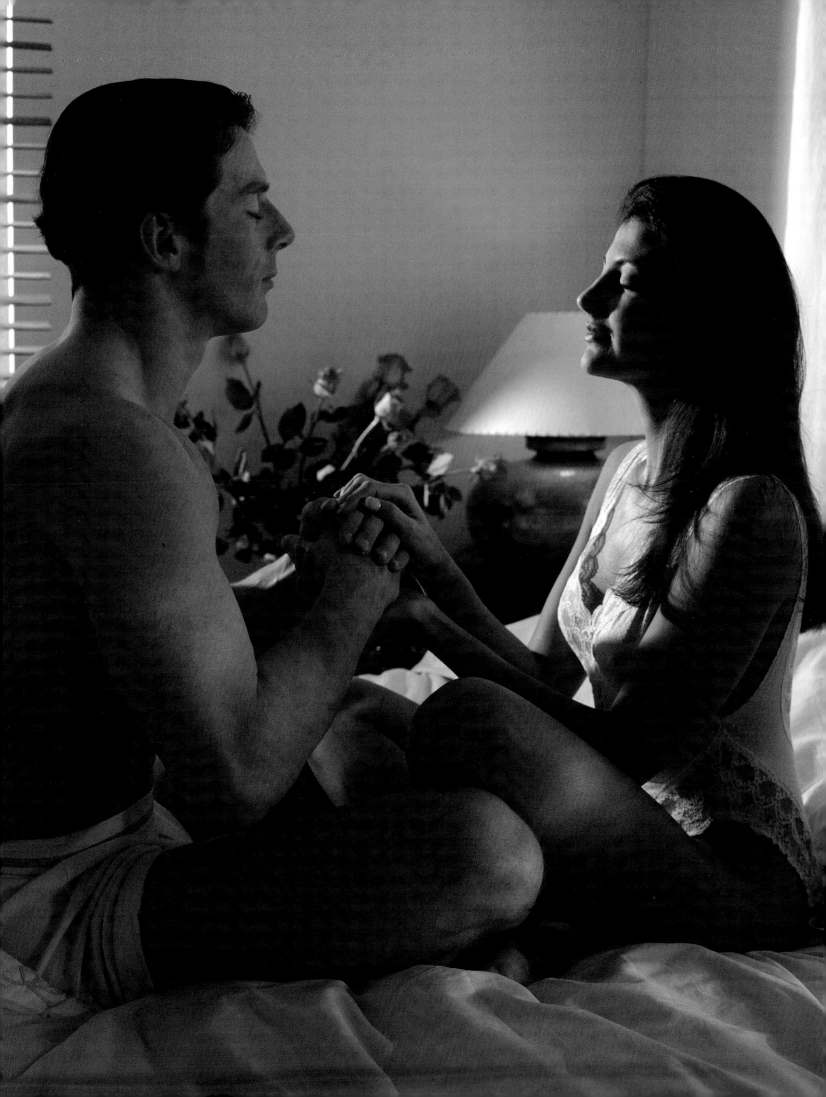

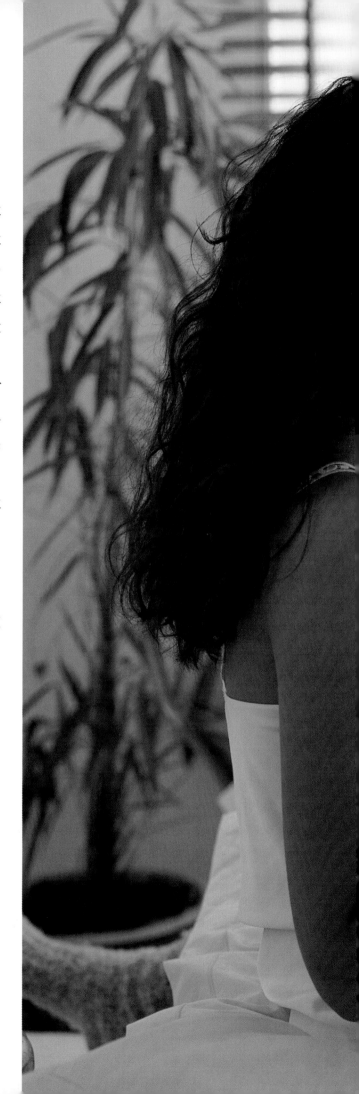

1 FIRST STEPS

Has the FUN gone out of your love-making? It is easy to let work, familiarity or parenthood dim the excitement of what used to be highly-charged sexual playtime. It is very easy to let physical intimacy wane almost without noticing. But getting warmth and eventually passion back into your sex lives cannot be achieved overnight. In some ways, you need to begin all over again, building up trust between each other and overcoming feelings of awkwardness and unease. A good starting place for your new, fun sex life is to notice what needs changing – and what doesn't. Real long-term solutions can only be found in communication. Ask yourselves what else besides sex gives you so much free, fulfilling fun? And 'fun' is the key word here. For quite often when we do make time for love-making, we take it all too seriously. In today's fast-moving world, there is something couples should always remember… Make time to make love. And take time to make it FUN!

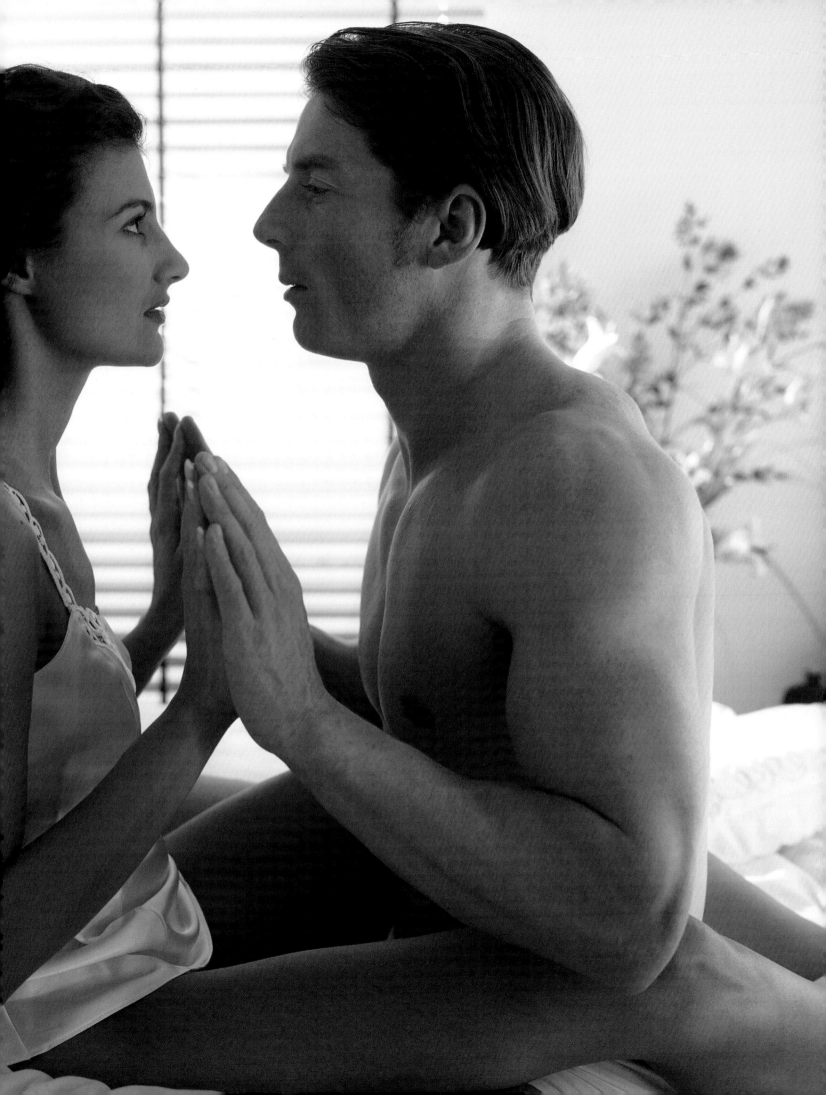

To keep alive that first spark of excitement that you felt during those early days of your relationship, one must remember to maintain a degree of romance, and to set time aside to enjoy once again those intimate moments together.

Close your eyes. Now think back to the very first time you made love with your partner. Remember the anticipation and the excitement of his or her hands on your body, the feel of your lover's mouth on yours, the promise of love-making never experienced before, the newness of it all, and the intensity of sexual need and fulfilment. Was the sex raw and unbridled? Fast and furious? Slow and deeply sensual? Does the memory of those first exciting encounters stay with you? Above all, does the thought of it make you smile?

Now think what love-making is like now. Is it far less frequent? Lacking in passion? Do you still really turn each other on? How many times have you had a headache, felt too tired or simply had no desire to make love? Has that aching for sexual satisfaction long gone? In short, has the FUN gone out of your love-making?

Of course, it is very hard to sustain a sexual relationship of the level it had when you first met; when your bodies were new to each other and when each other's sexual techniques were an exquisite mystery waiting to be savoured. It is easy to let work, familiarity and parenthood change what used to be highly-charged sexual playtime into quick, dutiful sexual intercourse.

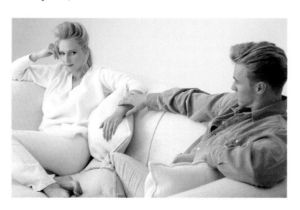

But nowadays, not having the time to recapture totally fulfilling and exciting love-making is not just an excuse wheeled out by long-term married couples. People in busy lifestyles don't have the time to spend on love-making that they should. This also applies to partners who are new to each other, whatever their age. Whether you are an aspiring high-flier working long hours or in middle-age and feeling insecure, love-making often takes a back seat. And quite often when we do make time, we take it all too seriously.

In today's fast-moving world, there is something couples should always remember: MAKE TIME TO MAKE MAKING LOVE FUN.

For some, sex is a serious business, but they are happy with the satisfaction they get out of it. That's fine, for satisfaction is what it's all about. But it is a little sad when there is so

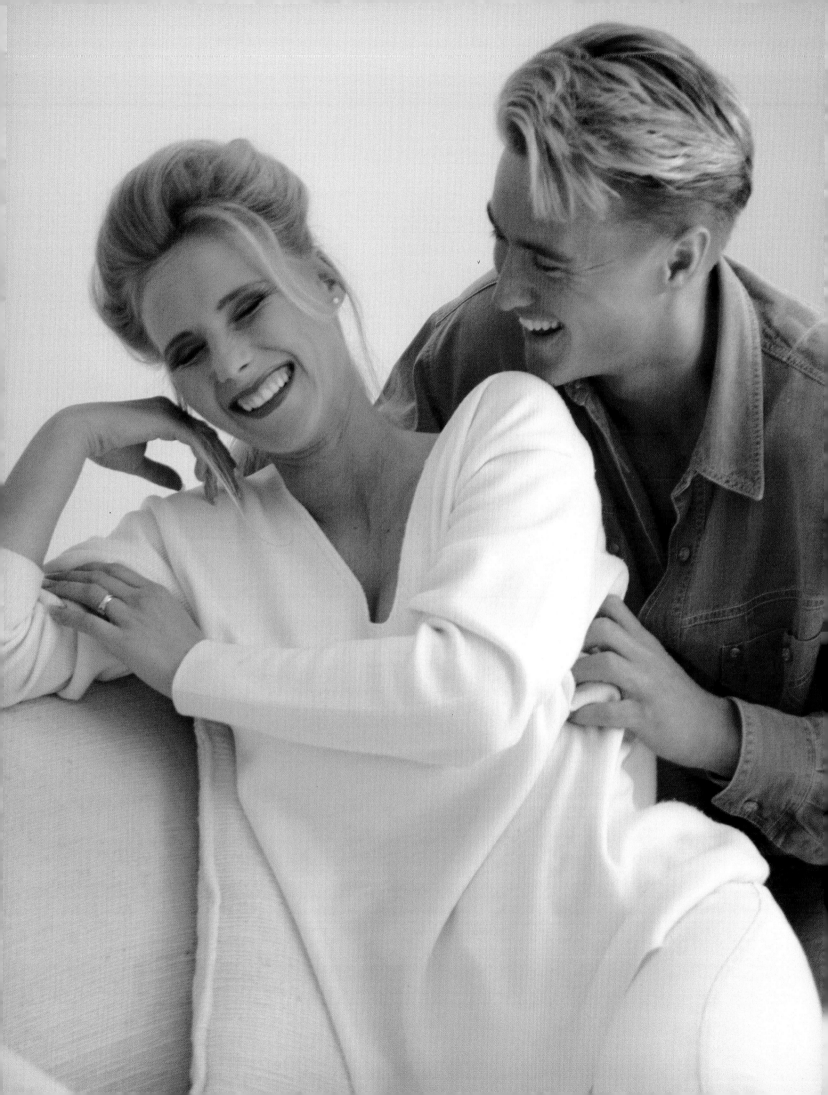

OPPOSITE: Foreplay is a crucial, sexual scene-setter.

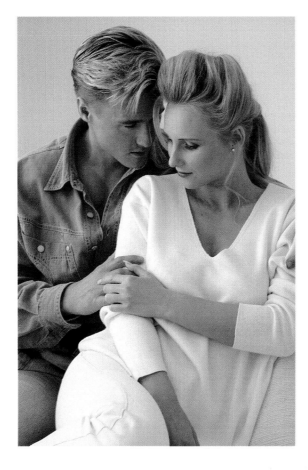

RIGHT: Fantasies should explore all your sexual thoughts and adventures.

RIGHT: Know the naughty and lovely ways to bring fun into your relationship.

their lives at all, not because they don't want it, but because, for various reasons, it is no longer an integral part of their relationship.

That is a dangerous situation to be in if you truly love your partner. He or she may not understand the reasons why you no longer want sexual contact and will be hurt that instead of feeling wanted, they simply feel invisible. It is a desperately sad situation when making love to that special person in your life becomes a chore on your list of 'things to do' rather than the ultimate way to express your feelings and make both your lives joyful and satisfying.

Not making love with the one you love is an abnormal state of affairs and completely undesirable. Making love with the one you love is natural, normal and utterly life-enhancing. There is no age limit to one's sex life and no rules or regulations.

Getting warmth and eventually passion back into your sex lives cannot be achieved overnight,

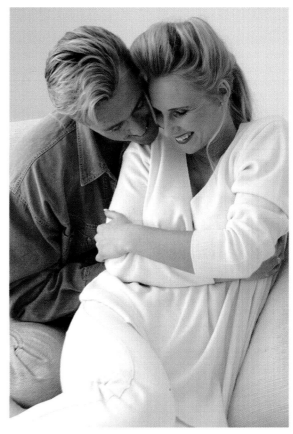

much more to be had from fun-time love-making. We're not talking about making it all one big joke or trivialising sex. Respect, trust and caring are just some of the ingredients necessary in any sexual relationship. It is true, too, that loving and laughter makes for satisfying sex – and puts the magic into any relationship. You may wonder what the point of having sex is, if you can't laugh and enjoy love. Who wants to feel *worse* and more miserable *after* love-making than *before*?

If you have allowed your sexual relationship to become dull and make love on a far less regular basis than you would like, you are probably craving the magic and sparkle you once knew. It is very easy to let physical intimacy wane, almost without noticing. First of all days pass without experiencing any sexual desire, then weeks. Often this turns into months. And there are couples for whom sex barely enters

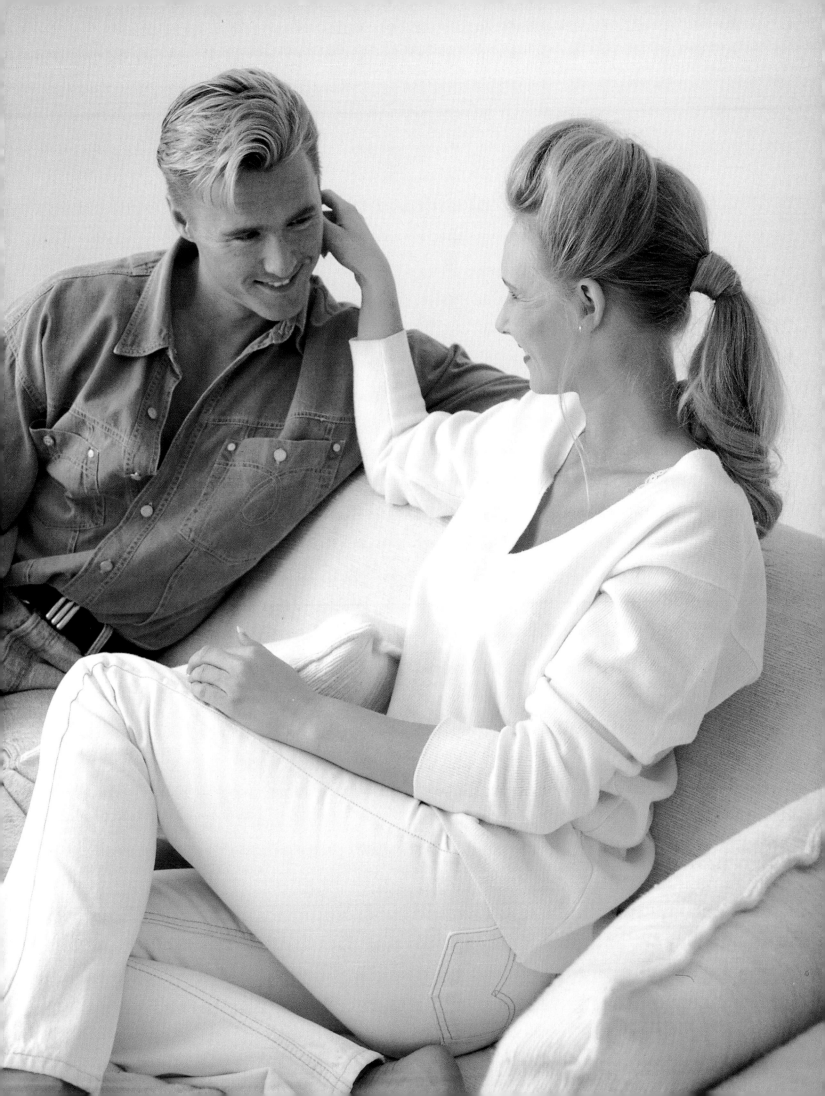

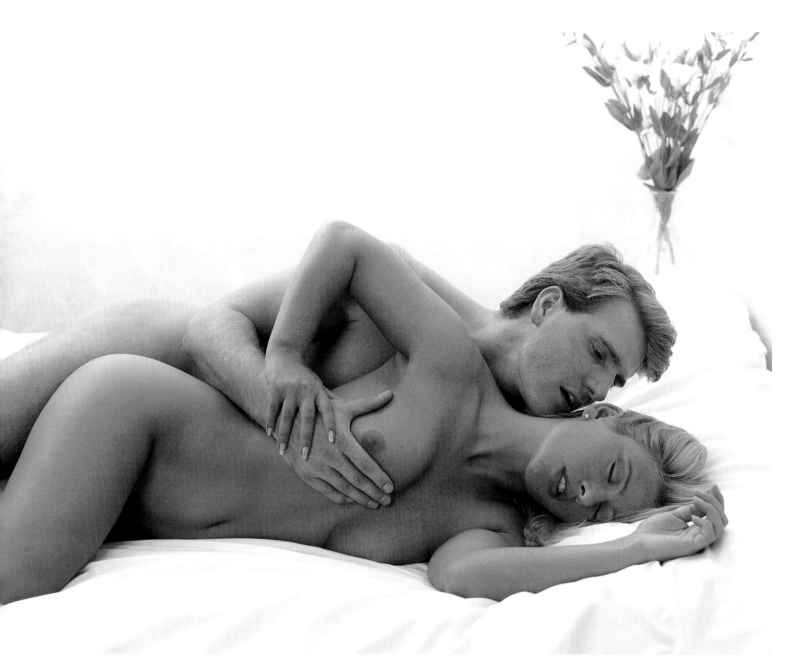

ABOVE: Guiding your partner's hands to your most sensual body parts will make sex more enjoyable for you both.

however. It involves starting all over again, building up trust between each other and overcoming feelings of awkwardness and unease. You may have forgotten how to talk dirty to each other – or perhaps you have always wanted to but never felt able. And there is no shame in being one of the scores of people who are just too embarrassed to talk in bed at all, let alone describe your favourite fantasies in detail or put into words how a particular activity makes you feel.

But you do need to know what you want in bed. It isn't a question of not feeling 'nice' by expressing secret desires. It is a simple matter of *enjoyment*.

A good starting place for your new, fun sex life is to notice what needs changing, and what doesn't. If your partner no longer responds in a positive or aroused way to something they used to obviously enjoy, there is absolutely no point in continuing that particular touch, position or movement. Perhaps they are bored with what they see as your carefully laid-out sexual performance timetable, unable to enjoy the immediate activity because they know exactly what's going to come next. Perhaps you have changed the way you carry out what was once so enjoyable. Perhaps you do not pay as much attention to your partner's responses. If this is so, change your ways!

If you feel awkward about what you see as 'admitting defeat' because something you thought was good enough no longer does the trick, make subtle changes. This could be moving hands, lips or tongue in a different way, at a different rhythm or at a different stage of your love-making. You don't need to announce you are trying something new, just quietly and gently try an alternative approach. Your partner's reaction should be enough to tell you that your new tactics have touched the spot.

Partners can be just as subtle in their encouragement of the changes taking place. They can gently guide hands or lips to the right place and at the right pace. A discreet movement of the body, murmur of enjoyment or positive response acknowledges that what is happening is pleasure-making or satisfying. There may even be occasions when sex becomes the best for a long time without either of you putting suggestions for change into words. But long-term solutions can only be found in communication, sexual freedom's best friend.

Relationships are nothing without commu-nication. And if you want your new-found

BELOW: Try using your lips on different areas of your partner's body; their response will let you know if it is pleasurable.

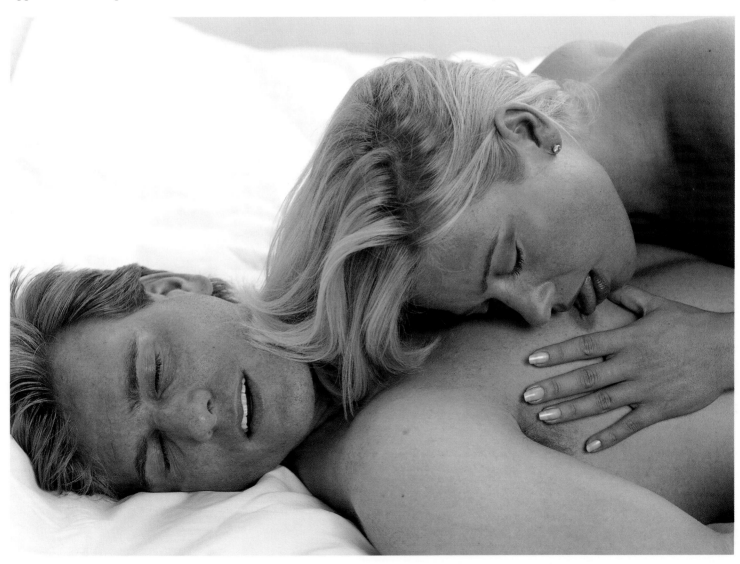

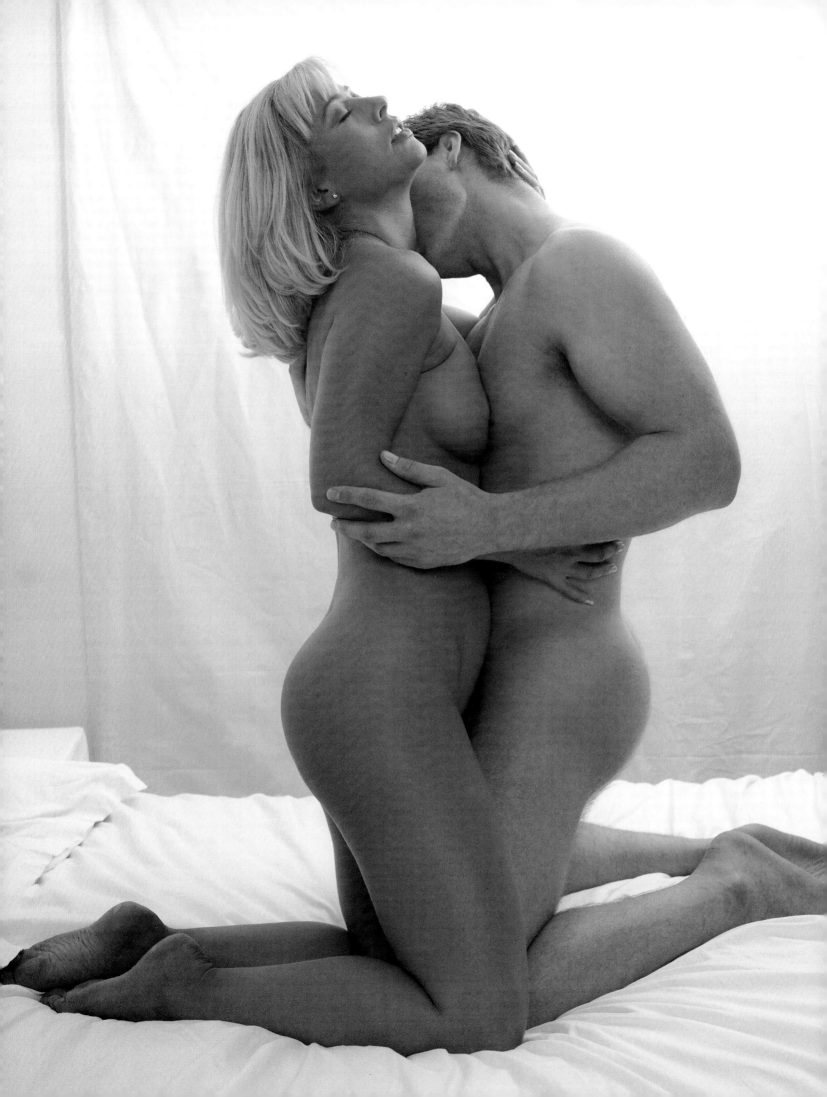

sexuality to continue you must promise yourself that there will be nothing on your mind to get in the way of relaxed love-making. How can anyone immerse themselves in physical pleasure when they are worried about an unwanted pregnancy, previous relationships or all the million other fears that take a second to creep in but can stay an awful lot longer? You and your partner need to talk about such worries and find mutually acceptable solutions wherever possible. It also helps to be honest with each other about everything, from feelings to more practical concerns. All of this clears the way for love-making with an uncluttered mind and thus a liberated body.

Once you feel comfortable with your partner, you will be able to discuss sexual wants as if you were simply discussing what to have for breakfast. Who knows? What you have felt shy of suggesting

all this time might be exactly what your partner has been desperate to do to you for months!

It is a case of taking the first step, taking a deep breath and boldly going where you have never gone before. And once you have expressed yourself in that initial, awkward first moment, that's the worst of it over! You will never feel that bad about feeling sexy ever again!

Talking about feelings, how do you feel about yourself? Do you dislike your body? Are there bits of it you feel don't match up to the stereotype of a sexually desirable human being? Do you believe that only a lithe, long-limbed god or goddess can enjoy sex and be sexually attractive? Do you worry about everything from a pimple on your chin to a wobbly tum preventing enjoyable sexual intercourse?

Think of all those women who, thanks to stereotyping, don't 'deserve' good sex because

OPPOSITE: Make an effort to get to know and feel at ease with each other's body.

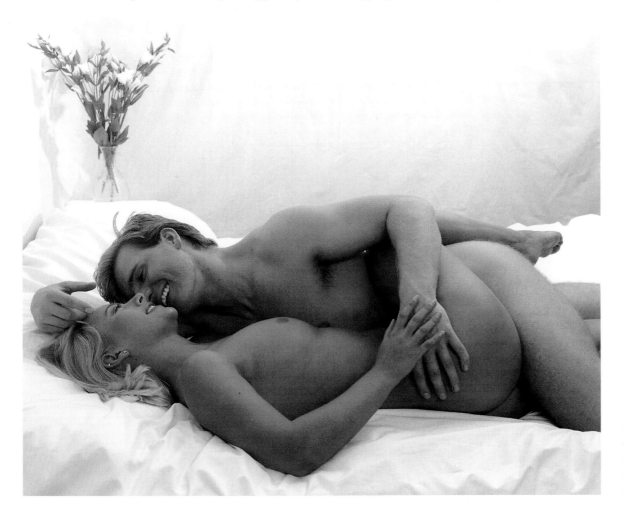

LEFT: Feeling comfortable with your body image will allow you to relax and enjoy uninhibited sex.

their breasts are too small or too large. Or because their bottoms are plumper than most. Or because their waist has expanded, their thighs are large, their hair brunette and not blonde... one could go on and on.

And how about the poor male? He lives in a world where, if we were foolish enough to believe it, erections come fast, furious and exceptionally frequently; where a climax is totally within his control; and where his partner begs an end to one explosive orgasm after another.

In truth, anyone, no matter what physical shortcomings they feel they have, has the right to enjoy sex. Satisfying sexual unions come from the desire and confidence to please – they have nothing to do with physical attributes.

By now, hopefully you are realising having sexual hang-ups is a bad thing. So, too, is denying yourself good love-making. Remember, sex is one of the few things to be enjoyed for free (in relationships anyway!) and in itself has no harmful effects. It is possible to have sex any

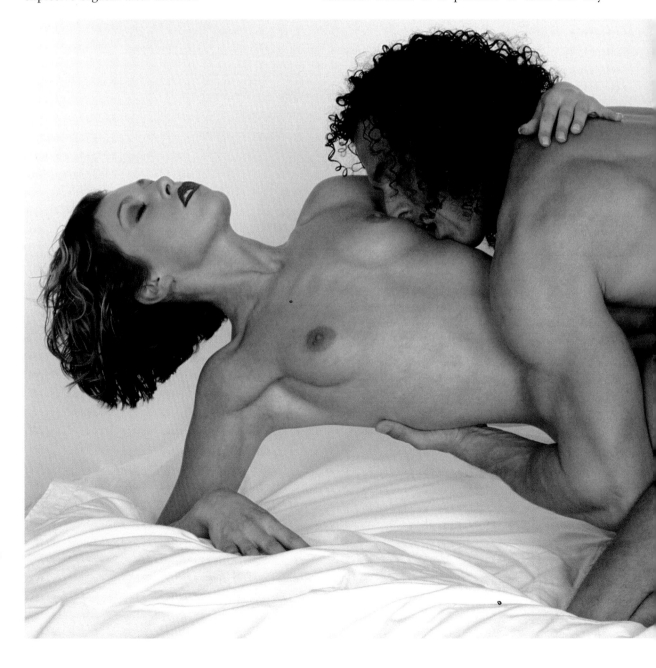

RIGHT: Sex should be a highly enjoyable experience for both partners; try to put the eroticism back into your lives.

moment of the day or night. So why do so many couples virtually set their watches by their sex sessions, even timing them for when their favourite television viewing is exhausted? Think of the pleasure you can have by choosing the best time for a prolonged and relaxed round of love-making or enjoying completely spontaneous sex out of 'normal hours'.

What else besides sex gives you so much free, fulfilling FUN? And fun is the key word here, for it's what this book is all about.

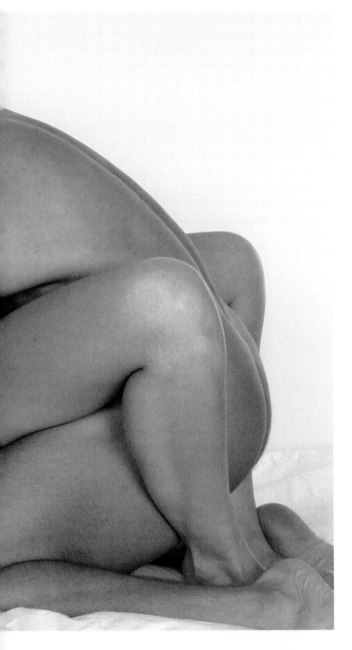

And before you put this book back on the shelf, thinking, 'Oh no, not another book about sex,' close your eyes again and think back to those first days of being together. It may be hard to remember now, but for you and your partner those days would indeed have been ones of sexual magic: learning what turns each other on, talking about each other's special desires and discovering new ways to please and tease without inhibition or embarrassment.

With human nature as quirky as it is, it is strange to ponder the fact that you are more likely to be adventurous and eager to please the first time you make love with someone than you are with a partner you have known for a while. Familiarity should never be the end of fun, especially when it comes to sexual matters.

The F-Plan of Sex

I'm sure you have heard of the F-Plan diet. Here's my F-Plan for bringing the sexual spark back into your relationship or igniting a new one. It ensures a healthy diet of loving sex – and a feast of good things for both of you.

Why F-Plan? Because of the five important ways you can bring the magic back to your sex life:
Foreplay a crucial sexual scene-setter with both mind and body aroused;
Fabulous Feelings to get you in the mood with tender touches and physical awareness;
Fantasies exploring the hidden depths of sexual thoughts and adventures and using them to get really turned on;
Fulfilment ensuring your love-making leaves you both with a feeling of total satisfaction;
And of course **Fun**, where you can learn about naughtily lovely ways to bring laughter and lust back into your lives.
This isn't just another sexual technique book. It's a book for people who want to bring sexy smiles back into their bedroom and laughter into their sex lives.

This is a book for fun-time lovers. And that means you.

2 FOREPLAY

It is easy to forget, in a well-worn relationship, what fun can be had out of love-making. Even new lovers often forget this essential lesson because of all the excitement of getting on with things. Surprisingly few women reach orgasm through penetration, so sex play is vital. And most men now appreciate that you need foreplay to be a sensitive and satisfying lover. The questions each of us must ask ourselves are… How many times today have we touched our partners in a reassuring or loving way? Where and how do we touch them when we go to bed? Is it always a prelude to love-making? Above all, do we truly value our partner's body? Answer those questions honestly and we will realise that spending time on foreplay not only improves a woman's sexual satisfaction but means a man gets more out of it as well.

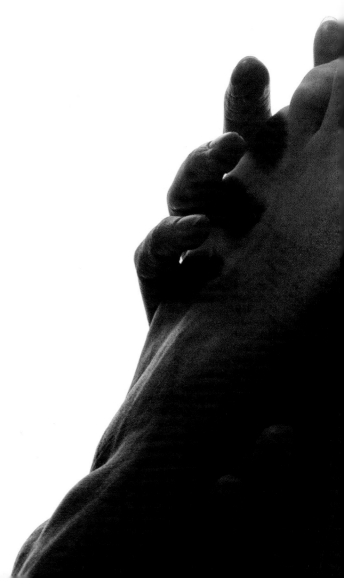

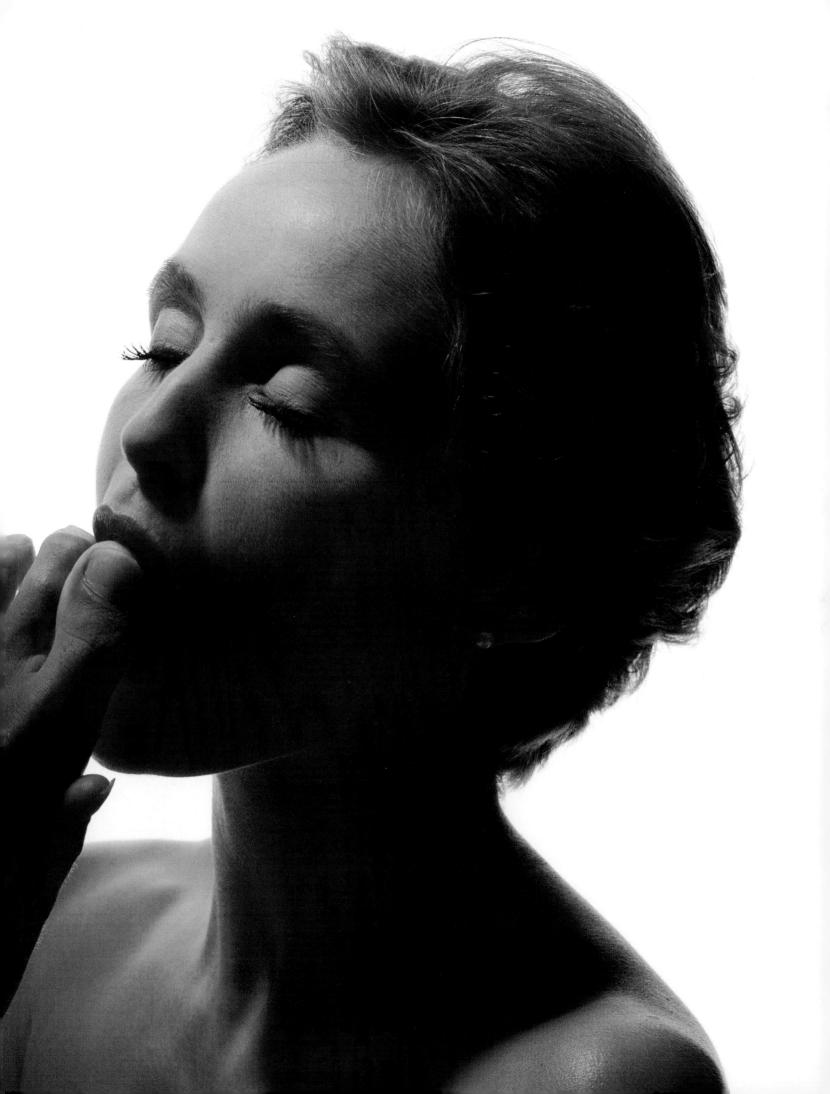

When you think about it, 'foreplay' is the least sexy word there is. It implies something you get over and done with before getting to playtime. But, by showing patience and sensitivity, one can derive enormous satisfaction and pleasure from it.

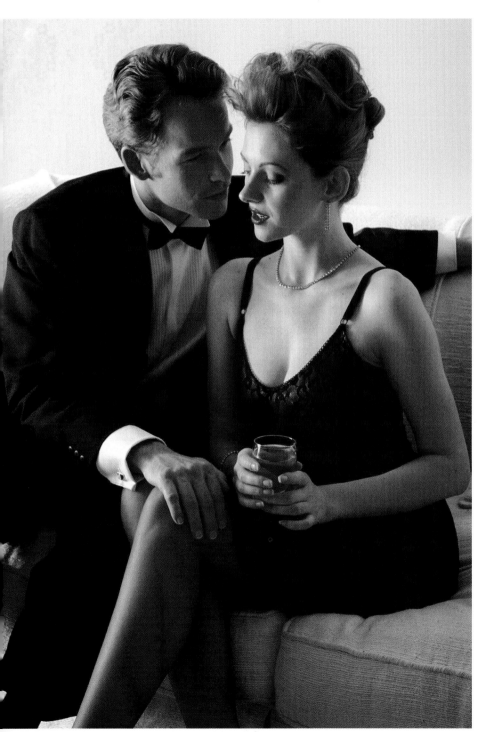

ABOVE: Getting passion back into your sex lives means building up trust.

Some people treat it as conveyor belt – never changing the order or even time spent on various bits of their partner's body. But if how, where and when you make love are important matters to consider, the quality of foreplay is crucial.

It is easy to forget, in a well-worn relationship, what fun a caress can be. And it is often disregarded in the beds of newly acquainted couples because of all the excitement of getting on with things. So it is no wonder that couples get bored with their sex lives when what should be prolonged, exciting and loving times become a basic act of penetration, with no thought or understanding of what should precede it. Yet surprisingly few women reach orgasm through penetration and most men desire some sex-play, two very good reasons why you need foreplay to be a sensitive and satisfying lover.

When sex becomes routine in a relationship, it is hard to believe that when the two of you first met, you were touching all the time. Think of all those light touches on the hand, on the back of the neck; all that stroking of hair, knees and backs. There were tongues in ears and brushing of lips, even in lighthearted conversations. Does that happen now?

How many times have you touched your partner in a reassuring or loving way today, for example? And where and how do you touch them when you go to bed? Is it always a prelude to love-making? Above all, do you value your partner's body? Do you worship it as part of sexual intercourse?

OPPOSITE: In a fast-moving world, our rule should be to make time to make love.

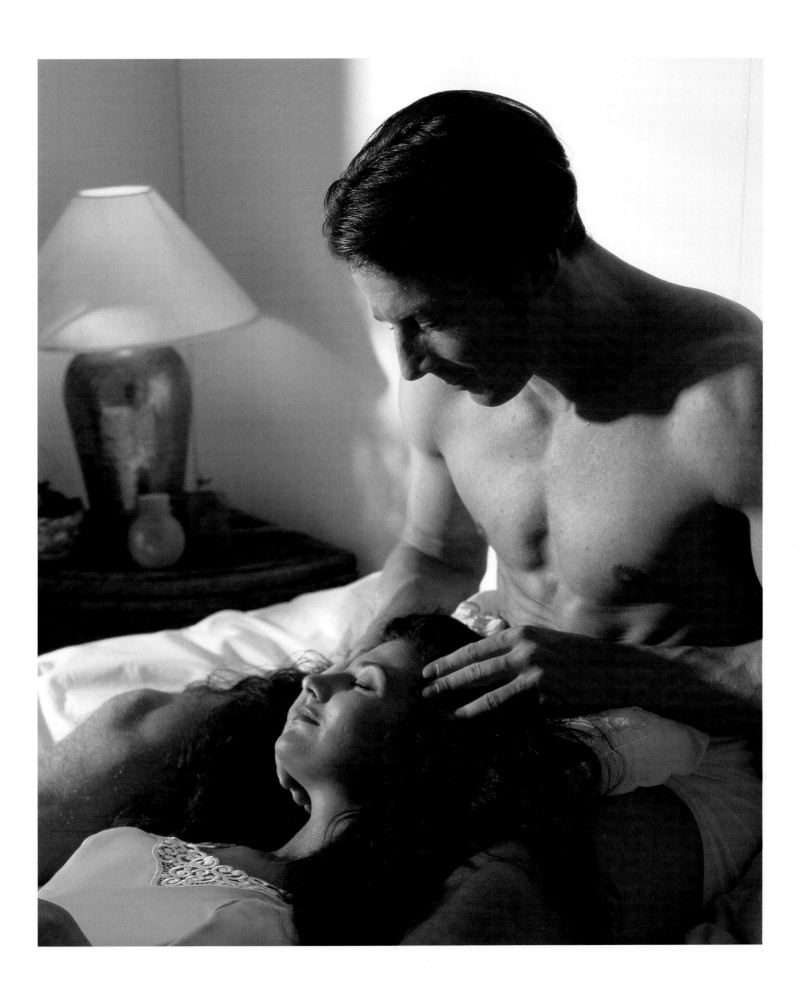

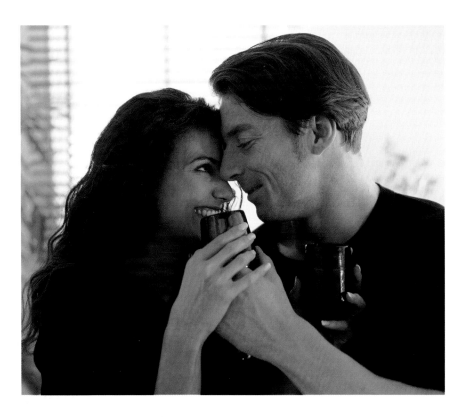

ABOVE: Close your eyes and think back to the very first time you made love with your partner.

Like all dissatisfaction in sexual matters, foreplay problems can be attributed to both sexes. Women complain that men do not spend enough time arousing them. Men complain that they always have to take the lead, women not realising they like to be stroked, kissed in unusual places and generally have their senses set alight. Spending time on foreplay not only improves a woman's sexual satisfaction but means the man gets more out of it as well.

Try this simple test to compare how your rather jaded foreplay compares to more aware foreplay: In a kitchen, with appliances noisily churning away, or in an office with phones ringing, caress the back of your arm with your hand while focusing on a specific problem which is bothering you, such as money, family affairs or job worries. Then find yourself a peaceful part of the house or a quiet corner somewhere else and caress your arm again. Close your eyes, relax and let your fantasies wander, focusing on your feelings all the time. Examine the difference! The touch is not different, but the way you experienced it is.

That's why massage is both so relaxing and so arousing. Using your fingers and tongue in creative ways can bring your partner to orgasm, especially if you talk as you 'work', telling your lover what you want to do to them, how desirable they are and how much you want them.

Then there is kissing. Again, think back to when you first met. Sometimes every sentence you uttered was punctuated with a kiss. When the two of you laughed you kissed. Sometimes you were desperate to make up after a quarrel just so you could kiss.

How does that compare with now? Do you still kiss every day, whether you make love or not? After a while, some couples even detach kissing from making love, concentrating instead on the actual act instead of true intimacy.

Perhaps kissing has become so familiar that it no longer turns you on. Perhaps you ought to change the way you kiss. Why not pretend you are kissing your partner for the very first time. Use nibbles. Use your tongue. Treat kissing as if it's the only way you can make love to your partner – and the only way to reach true sexual satisfaction. Spend time. Vary it. Be hard. Be soft. Be adventurous.

Women might like to know that men enjoy passionate kissing. Men should know that women need to be kissed.

Once you have put kissing on the mouth back into your love-making, move on to kissing the rest of your partner's body – every inch of it – again, as if the ultimate aim is to climax without penetration.

Kissing

Her to him: Women should use deep kisses to stimulate his lips, tongue and inside of his mouth. Flick your tongue in and out of his mouth and touch tongues. Arouse him by kissing the back of his neck, his ears and eyelids, progressing to his back, shoulders, nipples, stomach, inner thighs and genitals. Gentle biting and nibbling is welcome but not on his very sensitive areas.

Him to her: Eyelids are among her most sensitive areas. But don't forget tender kisses on the ears, neck and shoulders, moving all along the body to the feet. Take in inner arms and elbows, nipples, breasts (where many women enjoy gentle bites), tummy button and hips. Leave her special kissable bits until last.

Heightened fun can be added to foreplay with sex toys, but these shouldn't just be used on women – or to genital areas. They can be used to caress every part of the body to set nerves tingling – in the nicest way, of course!

Both sexes enjoy a vibrator against the ear lobes, lips, on the inside of the legs and around the anus and lower back.

Men might fancy having the length of the vibrator passed against the shaft of the penis, or the tip passed against the glans. They may also find it arousing to have the tip pressed against the scrotum and against the perineum (the skin immediately behind it).

Vibrators do not have to be inserted into the vagina. Women love having their labia and clitoris caressed with a vibrator. Some women might like

BELOW: Try kissing less obvious areas to make foreplay more adventurous.

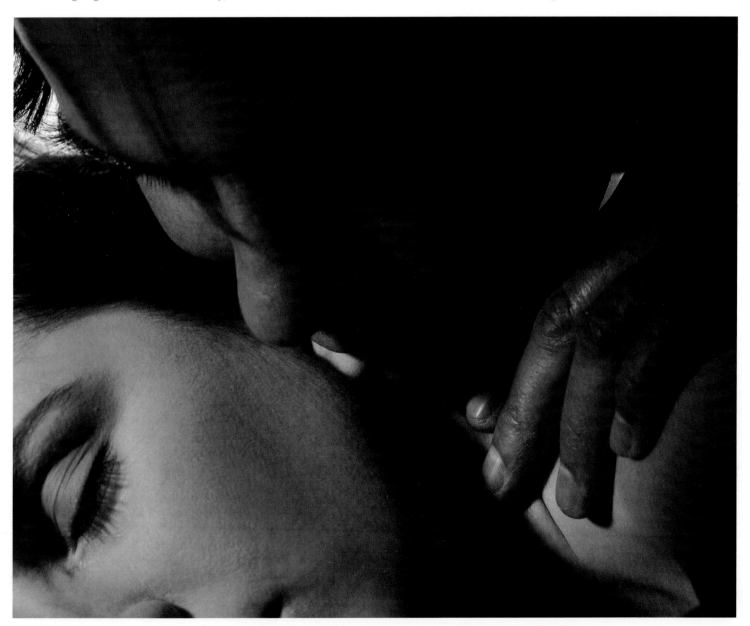

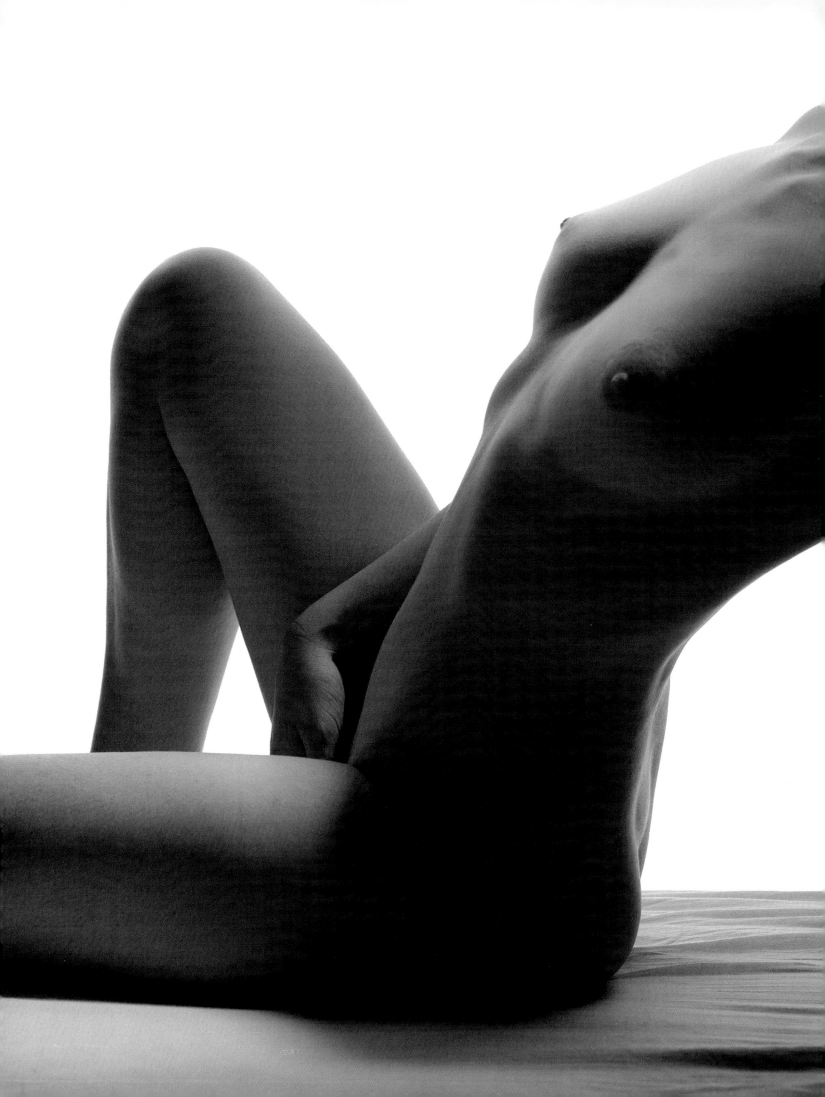

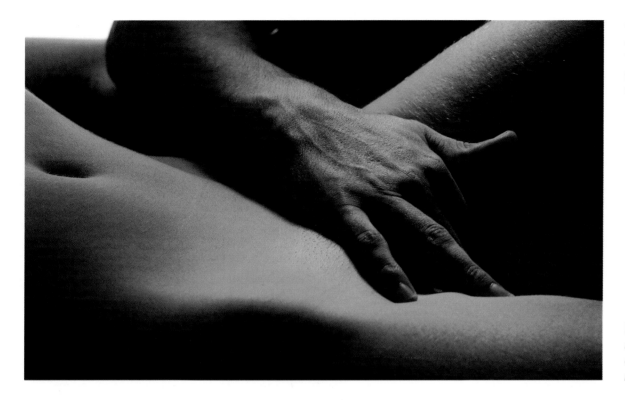

OPPOSITE:
Masturbation or
"solo sex" can be a
pleasurable prelude
to love-making.

LEFT: Perform
masturbation on each
other and find out what
really turns you on.

'rough play' with their sex toy, meaning faster or stronger use of a vibrator or dildo. She may even prefer to show off her sexual confidence by using such a toy on herself. Deeply satisfying to her, because she can control arousal exactly, and a big turn-on for the watching partner.

Why not play your own version of Pass The Parcel, only using a vibrator? One of you starts by passing it over your body, avoiding obvious areas such as nipples and genitals. Then do it again, only this time press harder. Increase the speed and do it again. Then pass the vibrator to your partner so they can do exactly the same. Next have your partner perform this highly pleasurable exercise on you. And you do the same to your partner. Or you might like to combine both your skills! She might have control of the apparatus, but you can take charge at the same time with your tongue and fingers. Enough to make any woman surrender and you haven't even got to 'full sex' yet!

Masturbation does not have to be enjoyed alone, even if it is nicknamed 'solo sex'. It is something you can do to each other or yourself while you partner watches. There is much to be learned by masturbating, whether alone or with

your lover. You can discover what turns you on and pass on the good news to your partner. There should certainly be no guilt attached to pleasuring yourself. Finding out what brings you to orgasm will obviously add to your love-making because knowing what pleases you will help your partner please you!

BELOW: Vibrators
can be a highly
effective way of
achieving maximum
self-satisfaction.

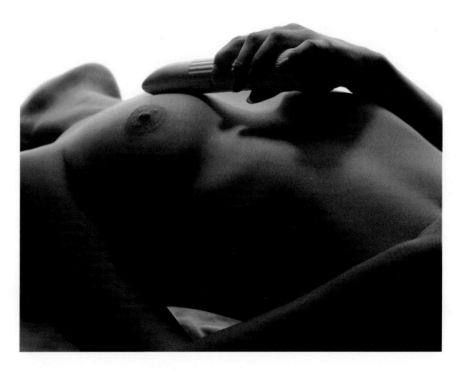

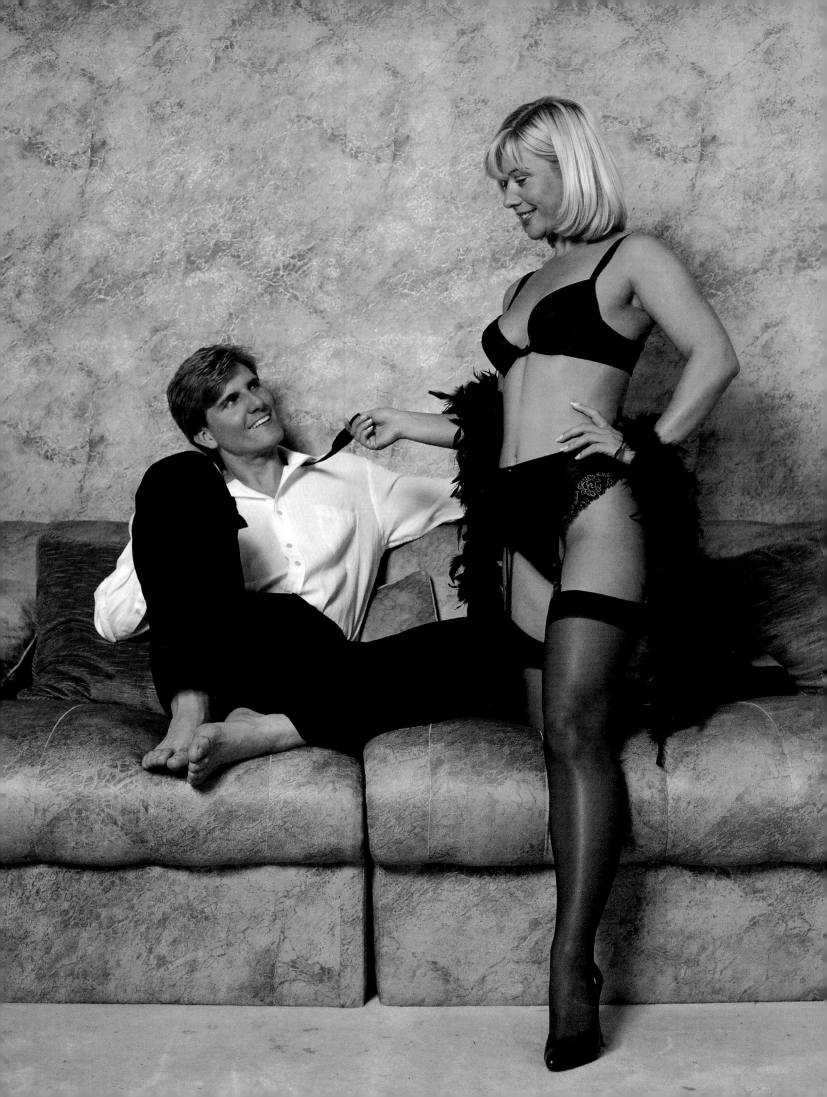

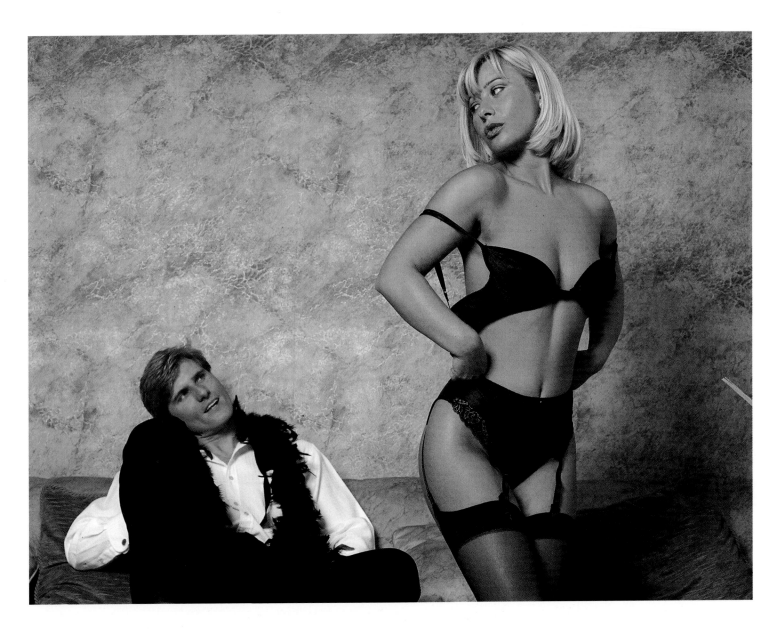

If either of you likes to fantasise, the masturbation part of sexual playtime is a good time to start. Encourage each other to describe your fantasies. Indulge in a little role-playing. Have fun with sexy pictures that come to mind and narrate your own stories of eroticism. Fantasising, as our chapter Fantasies shows, is an important part of satisfying sex. It is not just the one who is talking who gets aroused, but the listener, too.

Fantasies can transform simple masturbation into elaborate foreplay. They turn you on, prolong the excitement of love-making and often bring on orgasm before penetration. It is a good idea to 'rehearse' your fantasy in your mind several times

if you plan to run through it with your partner, so that everything is just perfect on your opening night! This could either be telling your own story or acting it out – as long as both of you are happy about doing this.

However, one fantasy that many men and women have is very straightforward: They want to see their partner taking off their clothes in a sexy and alluring way. Straightforward, yes; easily executed, no! Because of the many hang-ups we have about our bodies, we feel that no one wants to witness us getting undressed as a seriously sexual performance. It is one thing to pay to see professionals do it on stage, with their tanned torsos, tight tummies and skill at kicking off

ABOVE: Absorb yourself in the fantasy and enjoy!

OPPOSITE: Undressing sexily is just one way of achieving imaginative and adventurous foreplay.

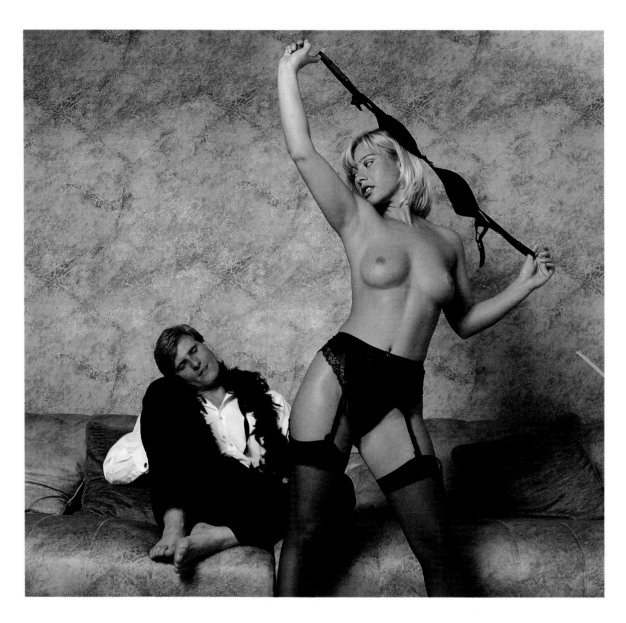

ABOVE: Slow and
sensual stripping will
result in great sexual
entertainment.

OPPOSITE: Don't
take it too seriously.
Both you and your
partner should enjoy
the experience.

knickers. But in the bedroom of a semi-detached, when you have just had a nasty shock on the bathroom scales, makes most of us feel totally inadequate and perfectly foolish. This doesn't have to be the case. You are loved for you and your body. If it can be pleasured and can please in bed, remember that's the same body you will be divesting of clothes as sexual entertainment for your partner.

Even if you have never thought of asking your partner to strip for you or if you have never done a strip for them, you are probably aware that how we undress can be a great prelude to making

love. Of course, the order in which you remove your clothes is important, especially in the knowledge that men leaving their socks until last is not a joke.

This may sound mundane, but here is the usual running order for stripping off for men and women: Men:- Jacket or sweater, shoes and socks, tie and shirt, trousers, pants. Women:- Jacket or sweater, shoes (and tights, if worn), blouse, skirt or trousers, stockings and suspenders (if preferred to tights), bra, knickers.

Stripping is best done slowly and sensuously – unless you're embarking on a fast and furious

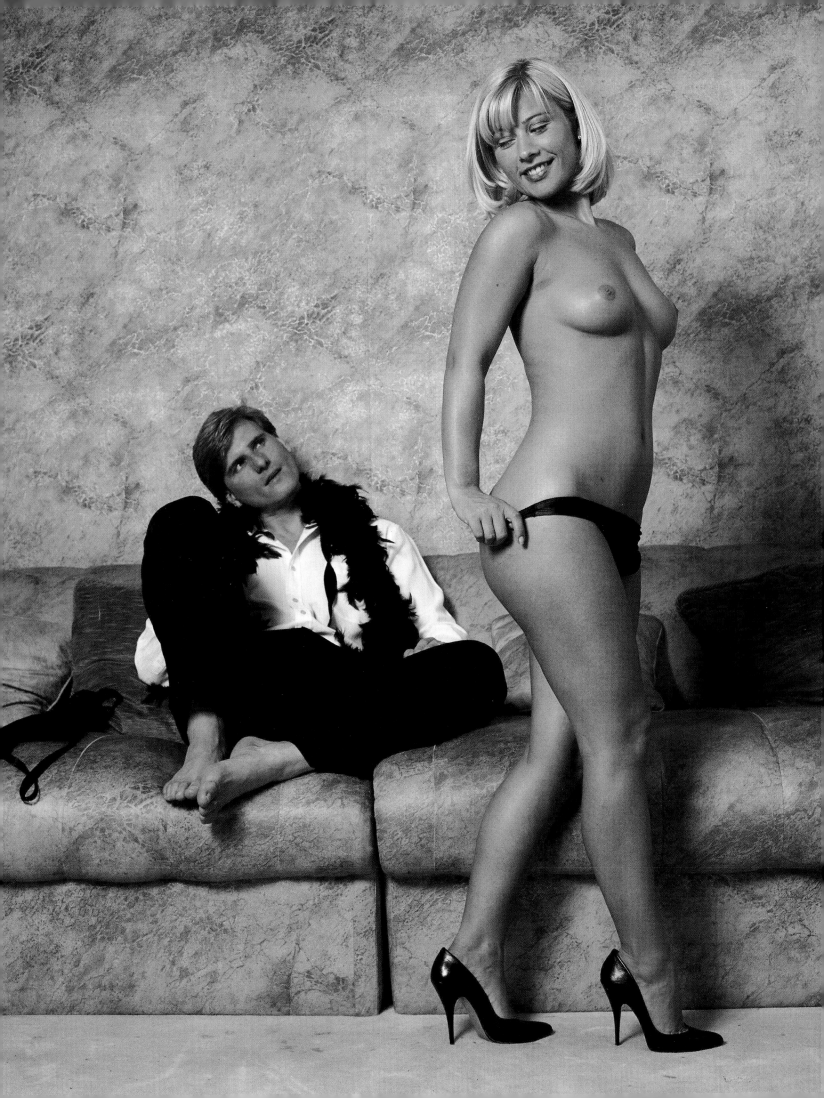

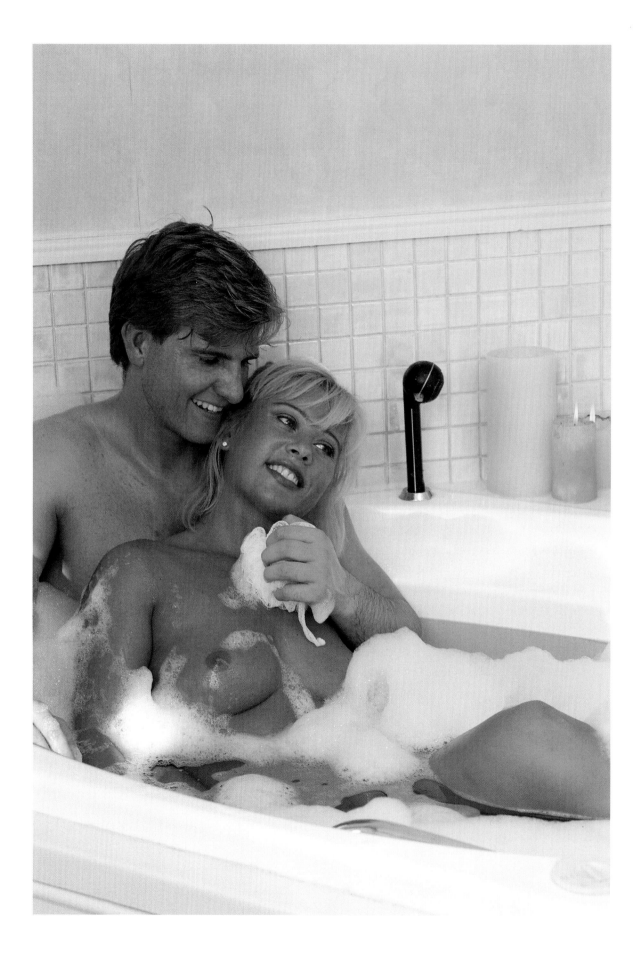

RIGHT: Get in the mood with a relaxing and scented bath.

'quickie' when neither cares how sexily buttons are undone! If you want to try it, make sure you have attractive if not sexy underwear on, dim the lights and imagine yourself performing for a crowd who find your every movement a massive turn-on. If it all goes horribly wrong and you trip over your knickers or there's hysterical laughter midway, don't despair. This book is all about having fun and if you both get the giggles at any time during sex-play, you simply laugh yourselves into bed. And you can't get better than that.

You might have realised that a lot of what enjoyably precedes full sex is visual stimulation or 'mental foreplay' – that is, pictures in your head. It is a myth that women are not as turned on by pornography as men. Both sexes like a bit of erotica to arouse them. Perhaps the main difference, however, is that far more women than men feel sexy after seeing the written word. They also often respond more to suggestion than the actual sex act. This is worth bearing in mind when beginning your new fun foreplay plans.

Men are a lot easier to get excited. Just the sight of a naked woman writhing around at a stag night strip show or in a video can get men hot under the collar. And there are shops and mail-order firms galore that sell 'specialist' films aimed at exciting you. Anyone who has seen one of these films knows that there is very little plot. No excuse is needed to be naked and there is a string of simulated sexual encounters. But some can be good fun to watch if you don't take them seriously and aren't expecting wonderful quality. The camera often focuses in close-up on pubic areas. It is only 'under the counter' films which allow erect penises to be shown. This 'harder' porn may or may not be to your taste.

The massive turnover in all sorts of sexually explicit videos is mainly down to men's predilections. But to be fair to the male sex, there are many who prefer their visual turn-ons to be

sexy and sensual rather than tacky titillation. So choose your videos with care to ensure that both of you not only feel aroused while watching them, but comfortable, too.

Feeling for Yourself

There are simple little ways you can get yourself in the mood for love-making:

For Her
- Sit on a soft blanket or bed cover in the nude. Feel the warm, cuddly sensations of the fabric
- Hold a satin cushion to your bosom and savour its cool, slithery surface
- Wear a fake fur coat inside out and enjoy the feel on your naked body
- Run a silky scarf across your legs and behind your knees
- Luxuriate in a bath full of bubbles

For Him
- Lie naked on the bed and visualise your own sexual paradise
- Be aware of your own skin – stroke it and imagine your hands are your partner's hands
- Apply your favourite aftershave or cologne in a gently, sensual way instead of just rubbing it on. Be aware of the sensation of the smell and feel of it
- Lie in a bath and isolate the many different sensations, such as the temperature of the water, the feel of soap, the slither of oil, the splashing from a tap
- Wrap yourself in a soft, warm dressing gown

For Both of You
- Bath together in scented and oiled water
- Use the oiliness to gently rub each other's skin
- Dry each other with soft, fluffy towels, stimulating your skin until the nerve endings are tingling
- Tickle each other with splashes of scented lotion or cologne. Your skin should now be wildly aware of the other skin so close to yours...

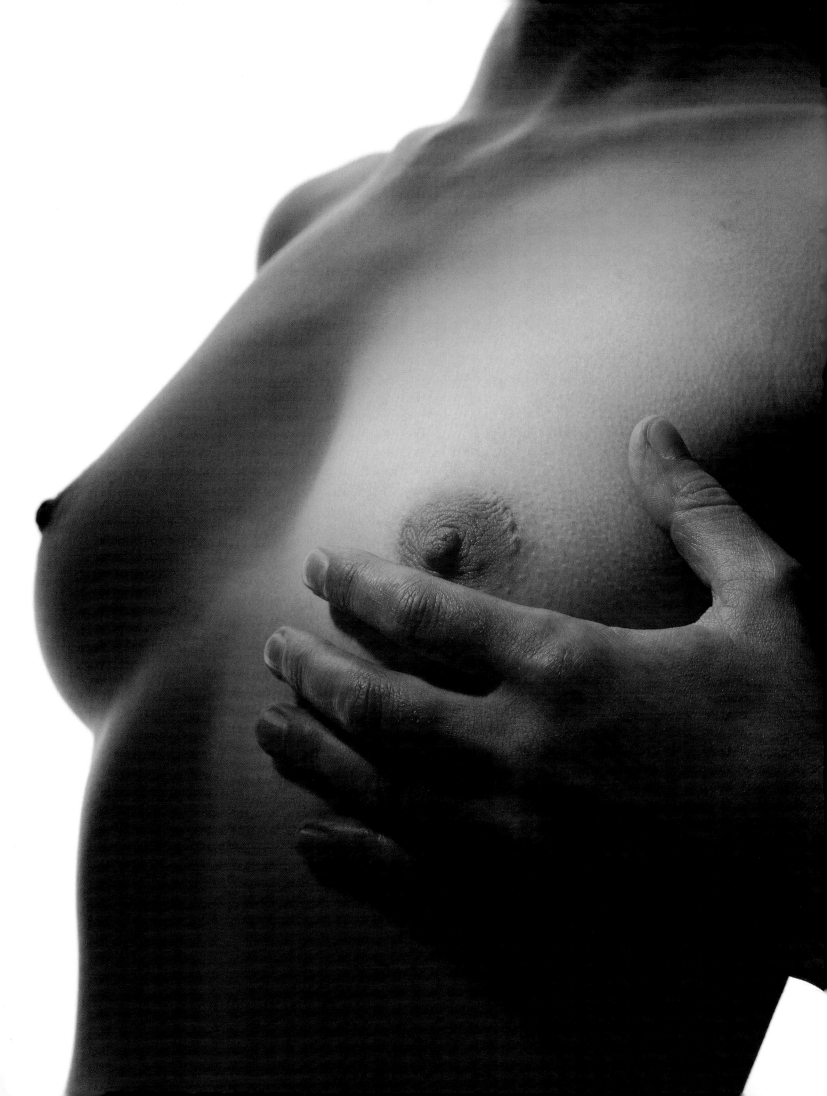

And what about touching? As we have seen above, it is easy to forget about the importance of non-penetrative physical contact. So here is where you start again.

Make sure you and your partner won't be disturbed (and definitely take the phone off the hook – who wants a third party chatting away on the answerphone?) and ensure that your bedroom is warm.

Now is the time to take it in turns simply touching each other. Let your partner touch you everywhere over your naked body, except the areas you would normally come into contact with during sex. The person being touched is not allowed to touch the other or allowed to speak. Instead, use your hand to guide the touching hand away if you are not enjoying the sensation. At first your partner may feel they are getting it all wrong, but eventually will realise the only experience you are having is one of total pleasure.

It is better to have your eyes closed throughout this touching 'lesson' so that you can focus totally on what you feel.

The even better news for the person being touched is that they get to control just how long their exquisite experience lasts! You can imagine how desperate the 'toucher' will be for their go. What you don't do is have intercourse, because the object of this sexy little game is to feel right and be totally aware of the importance of arousal before even contemplating penetration.

This has hopefully given you some idea of the importance of foreplay and the kind of things you can do before full sex. The main thing to remember is to linger over foreplay as long as possible. Two key phrases are:

Be inventive

Be attentive

And here you are, well on the way to understanding how much fun foreplay can be – for both of you.

OPPOSITE: Lingering touches will ensure heightened pleasure.

BELOW: Experiment by caressing areas of your partner's body you wouldn't usually touch.

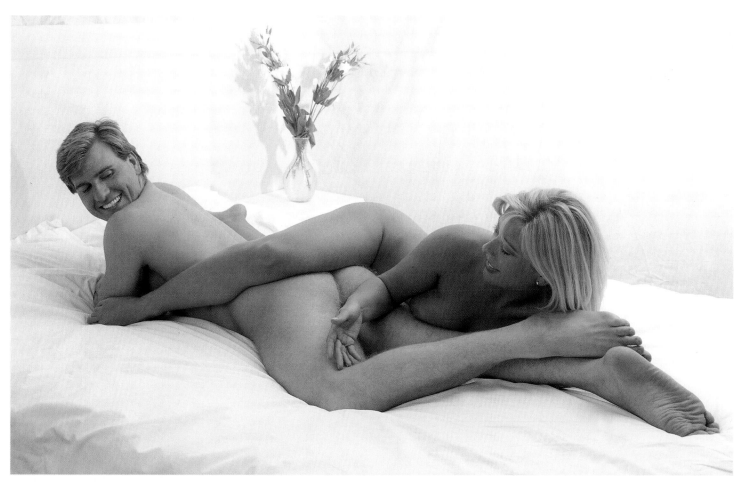

3 FABULOUS FEELINGS

Feeling fabulous and having 'Fabulous Feelings' are slightly different things. In this chapter, you will hopefully discover why you should enjoy both! You will learn how to experience various sensual experiences as you prepare for full skin-to-skin contact. You will discover the secrets of how to give each other full body massage using sexy oils – an essential guide to put you both in the mood for love, as well as easing tension and stress, crucial to make you feel completely relaxed. You will learn how aromatherapy and its magical scents can either help put the zing back into your sex life – or simply make you languidly loving!

Before you begin, there are several things you should do to create an atmosphere that is conducive to sensuality and awareness:

- Set the right mood. This means no interruptions, so take the telephone off the hook, lower the lights and light scented candles
- Ensure the room is at a comfortably warm temperature
- Put on some soothing music
- Prepare your 'working' surface by placing a blanket on the floor, bed or table
- If you want to use massage as a preliminary to love-making, you should both be naked
- Always warm the oils first
- At each new stage of the massage, pour liberal amounts of oil into your hands before applying them to your partner
- Try to keep one hand touching your lover as much as possible to give a feeling of continuity.

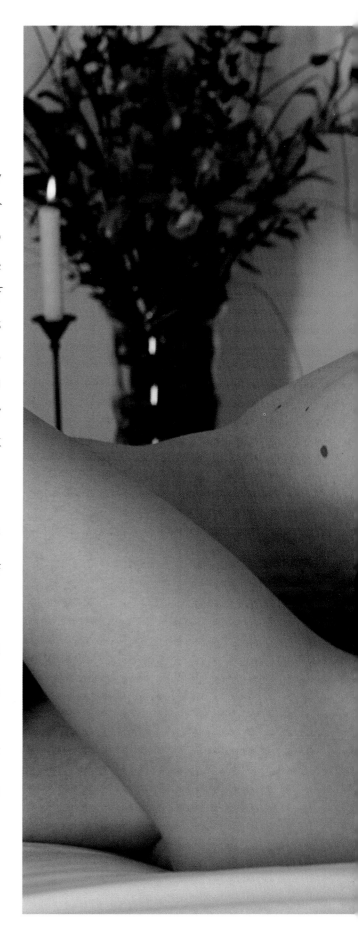

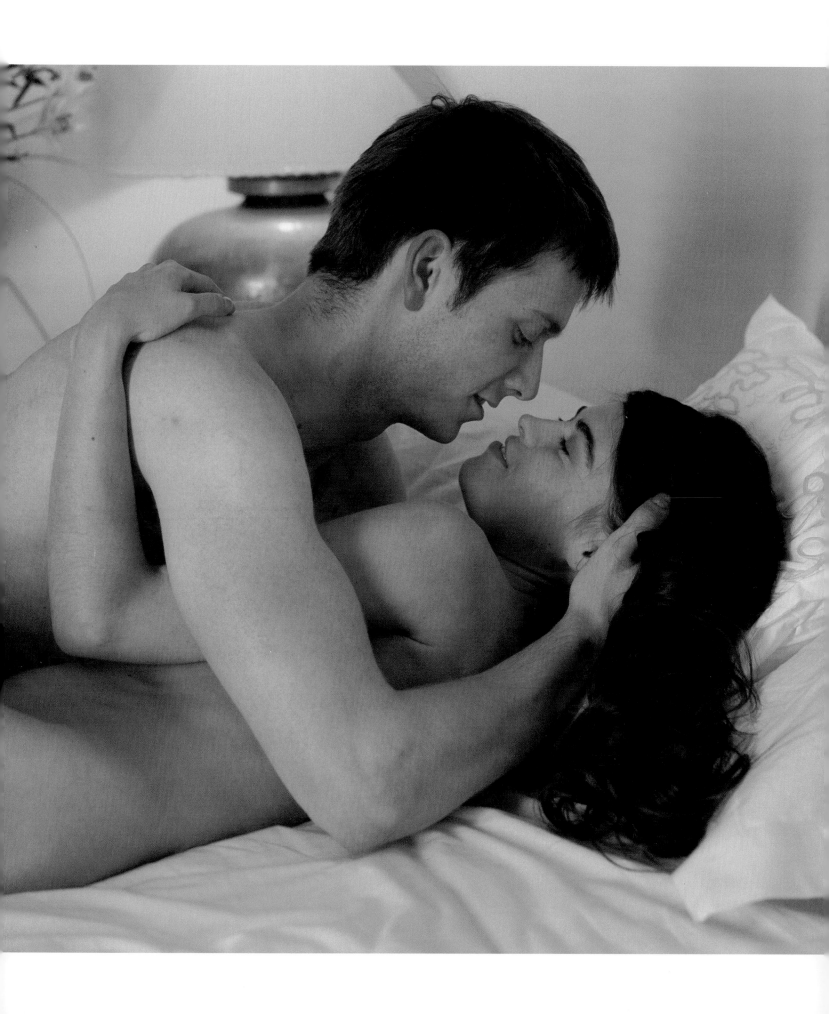

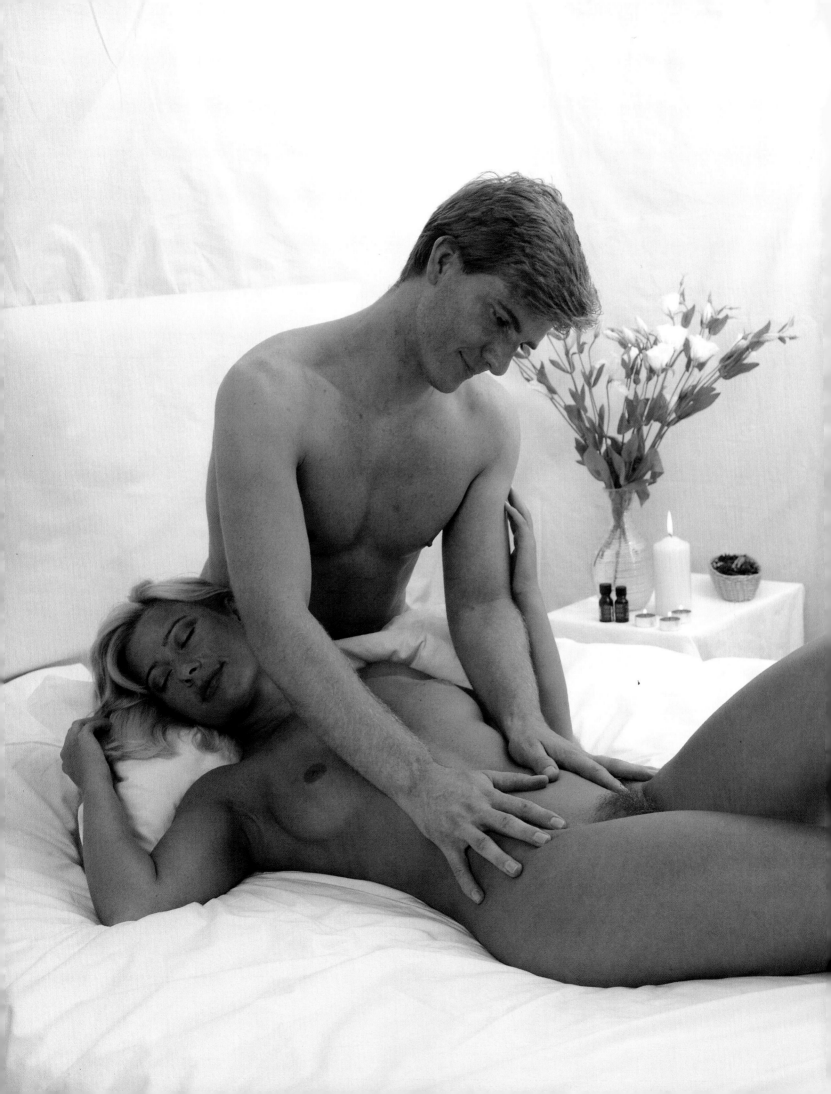

Mind and body are both involved in sex, which is why stress has such an effect on our love lives, causing conscious and unconscious tensions which inhibit physical and emotional relaxation between a couple. The pace of modern life does not always allow us the opportunity to discharge stress; instead, we hold it pent up within our bodies. If at the end of the day we feel tense, tired or anxious, we might view a partner's sexual desires as just one more unwanted demand on our time. Stress is one of the most common causes of impotence in men and lack of sexual response in women.

The solution to the problem is to avoid making it a problem in the first place. Learning the lessons of this chapter will make for a better sexual relationship and a better understanding of a loved one – back to body and mind!

Massage works on the whole person. It is fun to give and delightful to receive. It is perhaps the simplest of all therapies for stress. It is also one of the most beneficial – and probably the most pleasant. So learning to massage your partner as a therapy also equips you to perform some of the most exquisite exercises as a prelude to sex. It is rare that a treatment is also a sensuous pleasure!

You don't have to be qualified to give a relaxing massage. The very action of a loving touch soothes the mind and releases tensions in the body. The key is to allow plenty of time for it. Don't rush. Always start with a light touch. Light stroking of the skin has a direct effect on the nervous system.

Once your partner is at ease, firmer massage strokes can be employed to stretch the tissue and warm and relax tight, tense muscles. Performed softly, your strokes will relax; more vigorous and they can invigorate and stimulate and replenish vital energy.

OPPOSITE: Ease stress with a soothing massage using a light touch.

LEFT: Continue the massage with firmer strokes. This will serve to invigorate your partner.

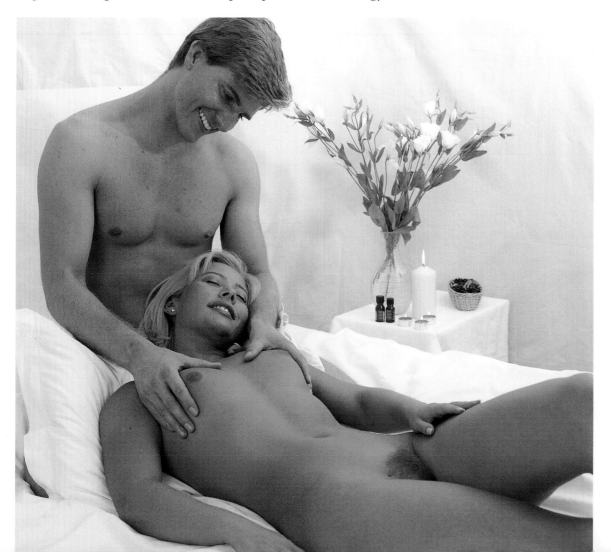

There are certain preludes to a sensual massage. When you arrange the location for your full massage session, the essentials are privacy, stillness, quietude and warmth. Ensure that you and your partner are positioned comfortably. The key, of course, is relaxation at all times.

Ideally you will also have found time to add to the delights of massage in other small but important ways....

You may first have freshened yourself with a shower – which, if taken together, is an enticing introduction to sexual massage. You should also have considered adding to the romance of the occasion by pandering to more senses than touch alone. Taste, sound and smell may also become elements of massage.

It's not suggested that you take a plate of sticky buns to your massage session, but the mood of relaxation is aided by a light meal beforehand – perhaps including foods that traditionally have aphrodisiac qualities, like oysters and chocolate. A bowl of exotic fruits, like mangoes and passion fruit, not only get the juices running down your chins but can trigger the sexual juices, too!

Sound is the second sense that can add to the enjoyment of massage. Soothing music is the perfect complement to sensual touch.

There is another prelude to massage that few people think of as sensual or loving. Few acts can convey love and respect for another person more than touching and massaging of the feet. Eastern cultures have always appreciated this

BELOW: Prior to massage stimulate the taste buds with aphrodisiac fruits.

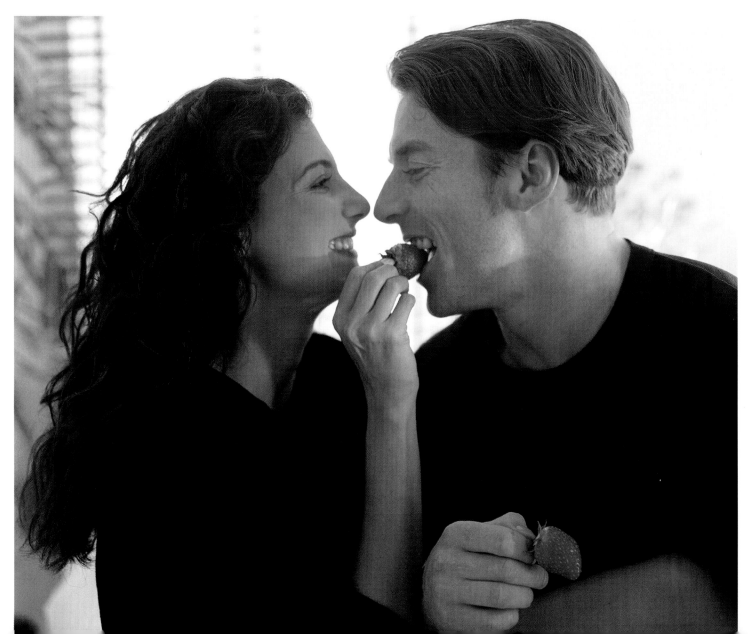

fact, though it seems to have become almost taboo in the West.

Preparing a foot bath, infused with steaming aromatic herbs and oils, can be the most unexpectedly pampering occasion. It not only invigorates the feet but is a restorative for tired, aching legs and indeed the whole body. In the East, you will be told that it also revives the spirit.

First prepare your partner for the experience. Seat him or her in a comfortable chair, place yourself on a footstool in front of them, and warm some towels on the radiator. It also helps if the lighting is as soft as the towels. Your actual foot bath should be wide enough for the feet to be flexed and the toes to move freely. Then fill it with warm water.

For a simple cleansing bath, add natural sea salt to the water and stir until the granules have dissolved. It not only cleans, of course, but also draws toxins out of the skin and relaxes the tissue. Simply flexing and unflexing the tendons will cause your partner to be swathed in a sensation of luxury. And that's using only salt!

For a more exotic, aromatic foot bath, you need some of the essential aromatherapy oils listed on the following pages. Carefully choose them to create the recipe which will induce the mood you wish to create. Only about five drops of oil in total should be needed for each footbath.

You can add to the aromatherapy oils on our list by seeking fresh ideas from the staff of your local health or beauty shop. Geranium and orange, for instance, are ideal ingredients for a footbath to invigorate your partner, whereas camomile and lavender aid relaxation.

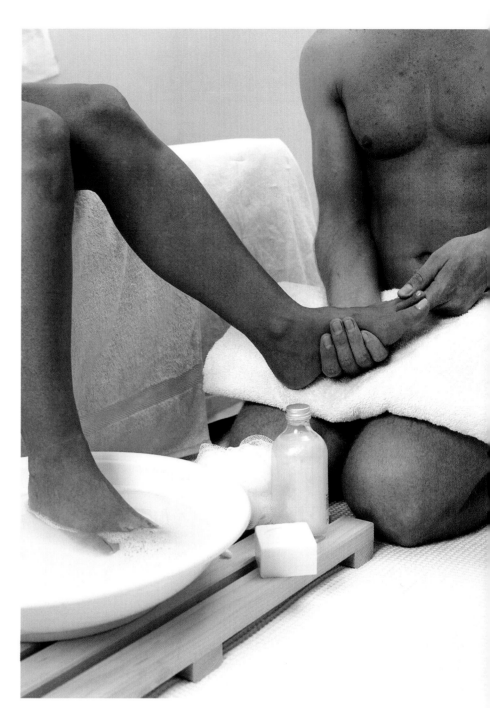

ABOVE: Pamper each other with a sensual and aromatic foot bath and massage.

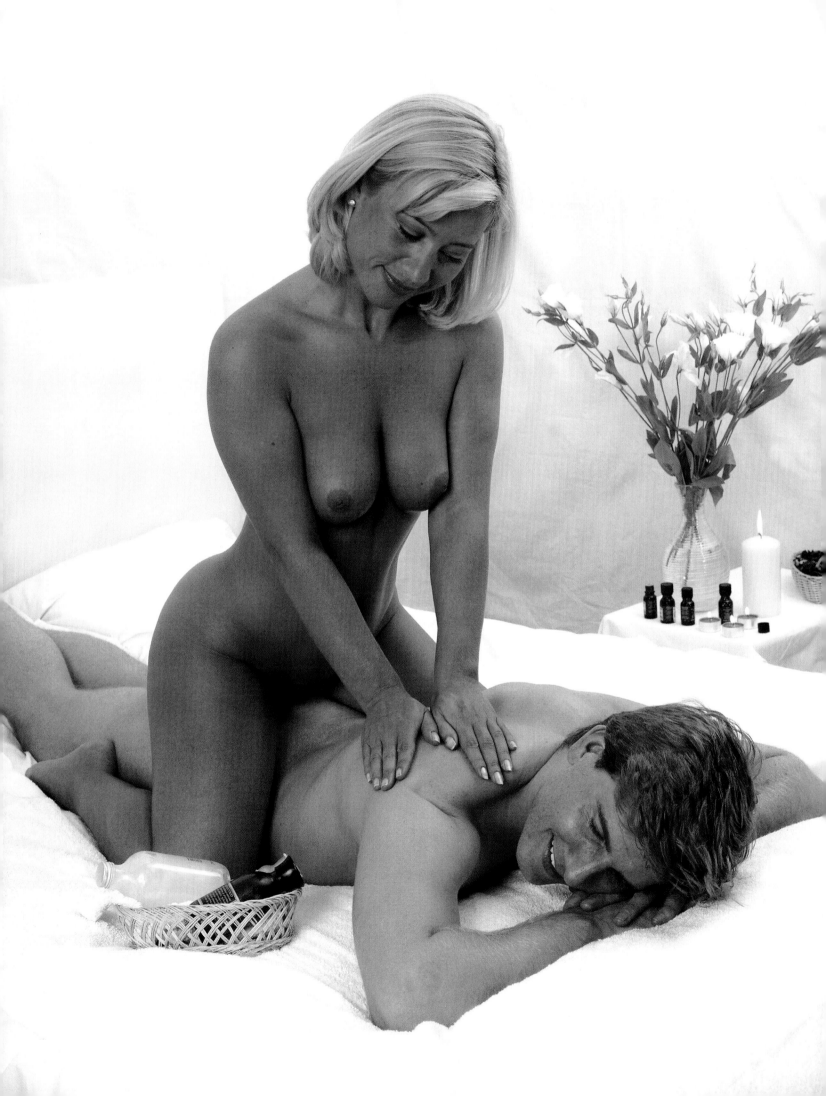

One of our senses – that of smell – is often forgotten as a means of enhancing eroticism in these modern times. Yet ancient apothecaries recognised that essential oils extracted from flowers, plants and herbs could be blended to highly potent effect. They have remedial properties which can beneficial to both body and emotions. Now aromatherapists are rediscovering these potions and blending them to create healthy recipes for romance.

Oil is a vital ingredient in massage, allowing you to lubricate the skin and give your strokes a sensuous feel. You can use baby oil purchased from a pharmacy or specially prepared massage oils from a health shop. But it can be an exciting challenge to prepare your own special recipe of oils.

If you are on a tight budget, choose a more common oil, such as lavender. The golden rule is that whatever oil you choose, ensure that it is pure. That goes for the vegetable oil to which you will probably be adding your aromatic oils.

To olive oil, grapeseed oil or other pure vegetable oil, add 10 to 15 drops of any mixture of the following....

Aromatherapy Oils

Bergamot is what gives Earl Grey tea its uniqueness. The delicate sweetness of the aroma is remarkable in that it both uplifts and relaxes. Stress sufferers should take note.

Black Pepper is revitalising and should keep a lover awake and energetic! Its sweet peppery aroma adds spice and vitality to love-making.

Cedarwood is the opposite of black pepper, relaxing the senses.

Frankincense concentrates the mind on the pleasures of the moment. This hauntingly spicy perfume clears the consciousness of niggling worries and replaces them with focused meditation.

Jasmine is a long-lingering, heady floral aroma. For would-be lovers who feel anxious or tense, it gives extra confidence. Its exotic aroma dissolves lethargy and heats the emotions.

Lavender is relaxing – but perhaps rather too lacking in excitement!

Lime is usually blended with other oils to add a light and playful energy, thanks to its bitter-sweet, mouth-watering smell.

Mandarin has a tangy citrus aroma which revitalises a flagging lover. It is a sure enhancer of youthfulness and vitality.

Melissa is soothing and calming.

Neroli has a haunting, bitter-sweet fragrance which evokes peaceful feelings while retaining an arousing effect.

Patchouli removes worries and replaces them with a meditative state of mind. But as well as calming the emotions, its musky and earthy aroma is a highly exotic ingredient.

Rose exudes a deeply luxuriant aroma which is uplifting and opens the heart to the tenderest feelings. Rose, it is claimed, alleviates sexual problems such as impotence and frigidity. In the past, it was used to treat women's reproductive disorders.

Rosewood has a woody yet floral fragrance which is highly seductive. It is calming yet uplifting and can help ease sexual anxiety.

Sandalwood is a masculine fragrance long attributed with aphrodisiac properties. The sweet, woody aroma certainly eases tension.

Ylang Ylang alleviates sexual tension by virtue of its sweet and heady floral fragrance. Anger dissolves and relaxation is aided.

OPPOSITE: Choose scented aromatherapy oils to enhance the eroticism of a massage.

BELOW: Once your partner is comfortable massage the areas that require most attention.

TOP RIGHT: Press the foot against your body and gently pull the toes.

BOTTOM RIGHT: Move your hands up over the calf to behind the knees.

Take turns in giving each other massage, focusing on the areas which require most attention. Start with your partner lying comfortably on his or her back. A rolled towel at the back of the neck will provide support. Try to keep one hand in contact with your lover as much as possible to give continuity. As you massage, try to keep your back straight and use the weight of your body to apply pressure.

Feet and Toes

With your partner lying face down, bend his or her leg at the knee. Cushion the foot against your body. Gently pull his toes. Place one hand flat across the top of the toes and with the other push firmly along the sole of the foot from toe to heel. With your thumbs, trace small circles along the top of the foot, from toes to ankle.

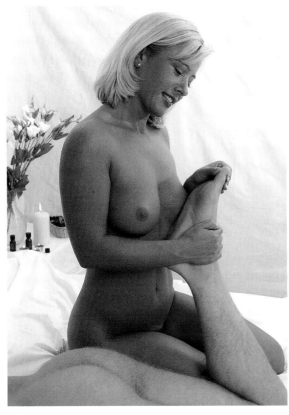

Legs and Knees

Your partner should be lying on his or her back. Kneel beside your partner, possibly straddling one leg. Cup your hands around the foot and move them up over the calf to behind the knee. Knees are highly sensitive so pause here and move your fingers in tight circles. Then continue your upward movement with your palms until they are either side of the thigh, moving up to the groin. Slide your hands gently back down the leg.

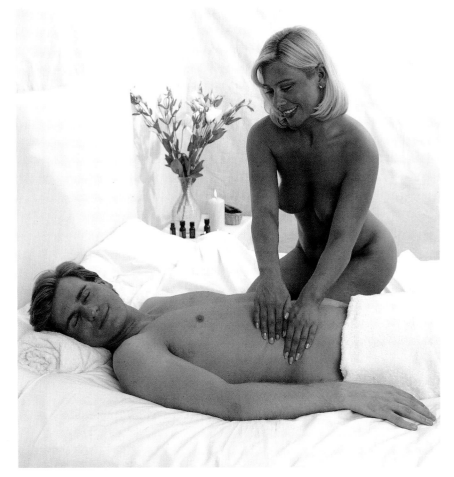

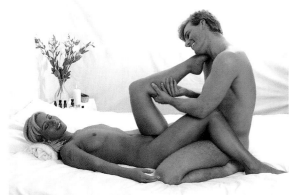

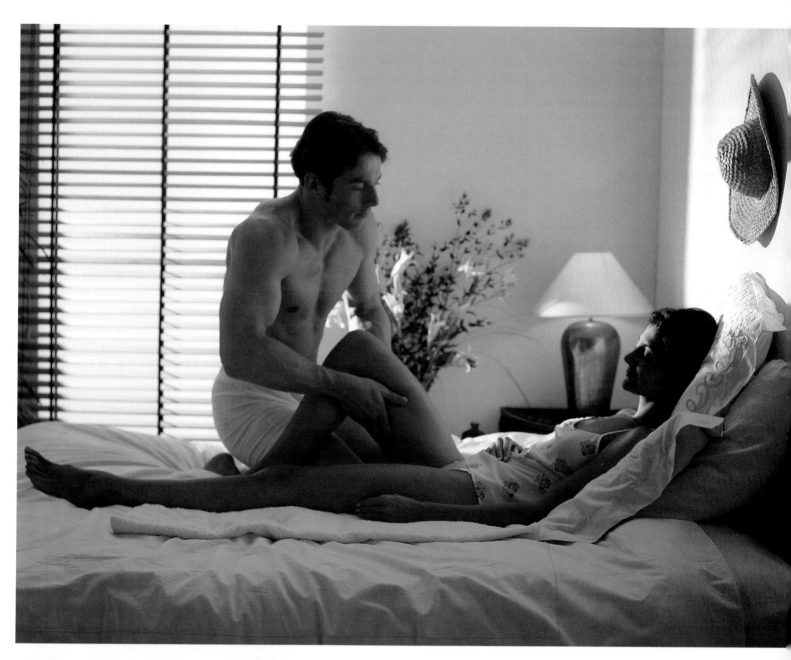

Buttocks

With your partner lying face down, straddle his or her thighs. Let your fingers trace the inside of the thighs before applying your palms to the cheeks of the buttocks. Use both hands to perform a kneading action on each buttock in turn. Scoop and squeeze the flesh in a continuous motion, back and forth. Buttocks store tension and deep massage of this area not only releases stresses but can relieve muscular pains.

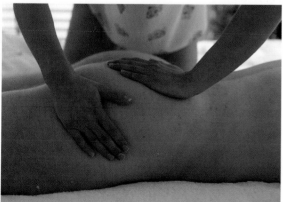

ABOVE: Place your palms at either side of the thigh moving up to the groin, then slide hands gently back down the leg.

LEFT: Apply palms to the cheeks of the buttocks with gentle pressure.

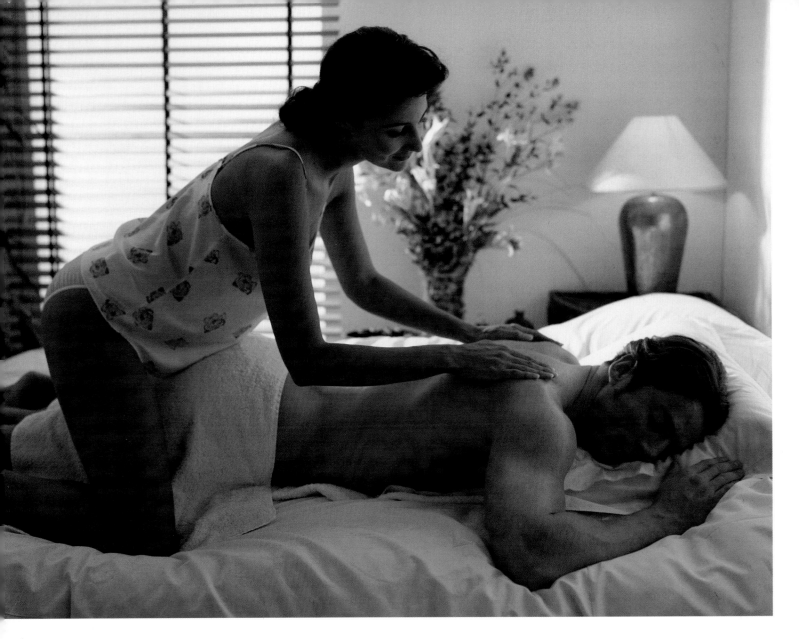

Back

Start at the base of the back, with hands either side of the spine. With palms flat, stroke upwards right to the top of the shoulders. Slide gently back then repeat the movement, moving further out from the spine each time so that you eventually cover the whole of the back.

Stomach

Ask your partner to roll over. With one hand on top of the other, use small circles to lightly move them across the stomach. Then place your hands either side of your lover's waist and gently slide them up and in towards the navel.

Hands and Arms

Open your lover's hand, palm upwards. Gently pull at each finger in turn. Using your thumbs, massage the surface of the palm of the hand with small circles. Next, with hands cupped, massage your partner's arms by stroking upwards from wrist to shoulder.

Shoulders

This is the commonest area of tension, so be prepared for some aches in the aftermath of a massage. Using your thumbs, make small circles along the muscles behind the top of the shoulders, then work inwards, towards the neck, using deep pressure. Slide your thumbs gently back. If the muscles you have been treating feel uncomfortable afterwards, fear not – this is a good sign and shows that your massage is working to loosen muscle tissue.

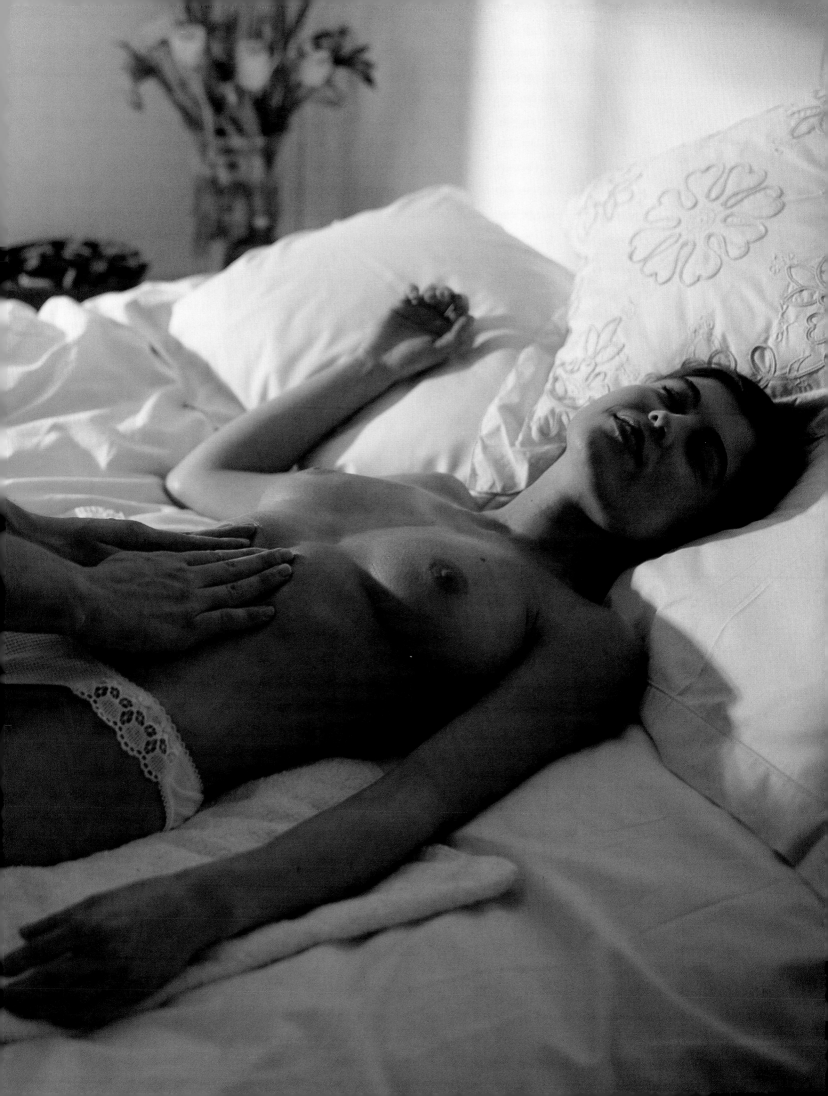

4 FANTASIES

Many people are ashamed of their sexual daydreams, yet they are no different to the type of daydreams lovers have all around the world. Fantasising is not being selfish with your partner – it is the opposite; wanting to please him or her while being pleasured yourself. Fantasies should be seen as nothing more than an elaborate daydream and, when of a sexual nature, nothing to be ashamed of. They are a sign of a healthy and fertile imagination. And living out those fantasies can bring new and enormously fulfilling dimensions to any relationship. There may be some fantasies you want to keep to yourself but many others that will be bettered by sharing. You just need the courage to talk to your partner about what fantasies really turn you on. That way, fantasy sex should be fantastic fun for both of you!

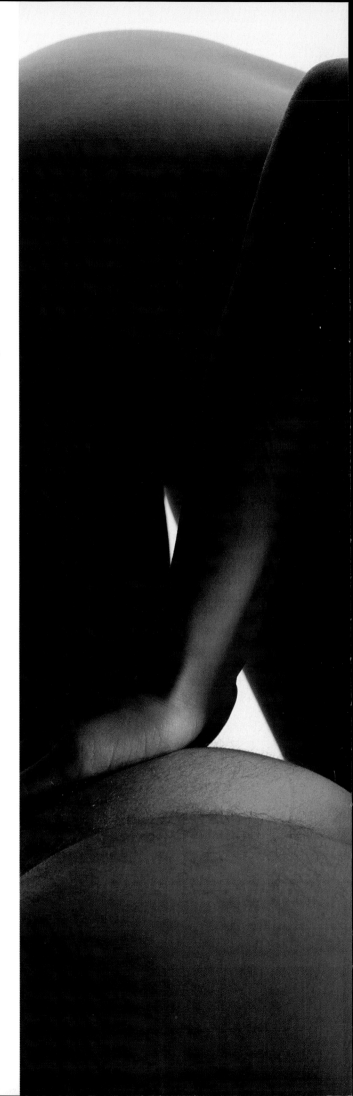

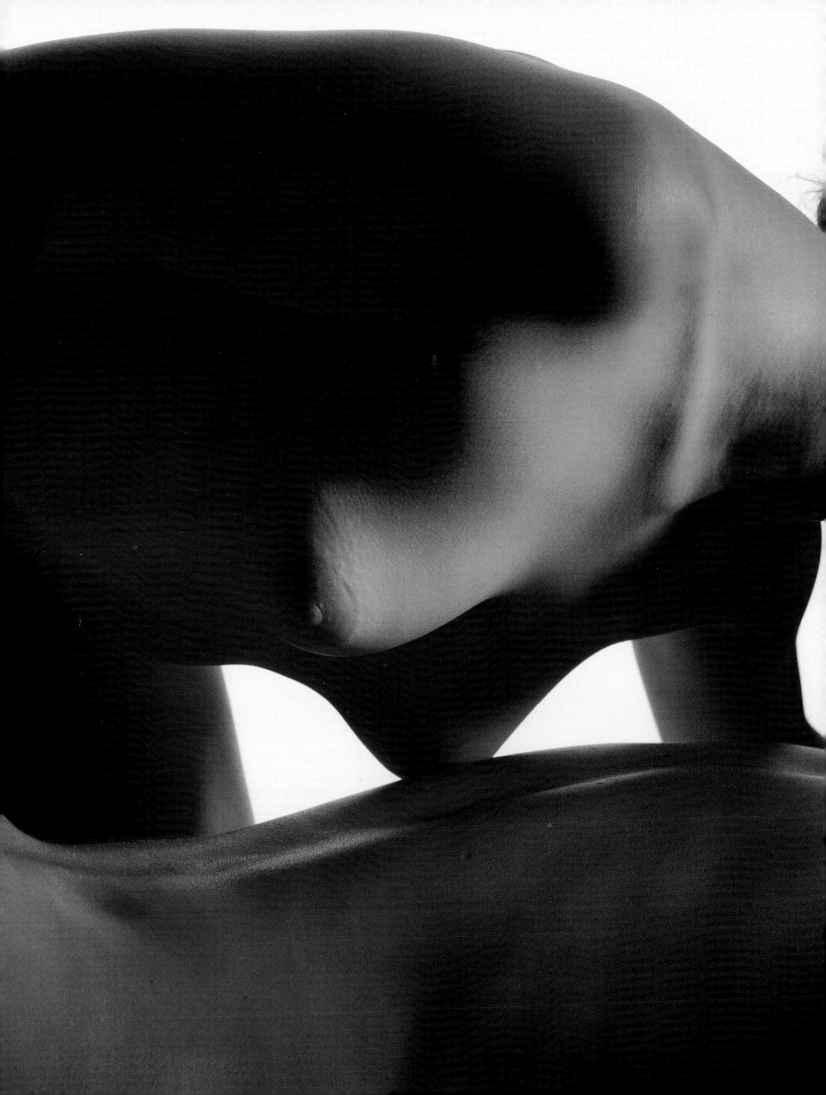

Not everyone will admit to it, but we all have sexual fantasies. They can be simple and straightforward, such as imagining making love with someone famous, or more adventurous such as having sex with a stranger or more than one person. If we were brave enough to talk about our secret fantasies, it is highly likely that they would be far more detailed and extraordinary than anything we have read in even the raunchiest of novels!

BELOW: Those who have the most developed fantasies also have the most athletic bedtimes.

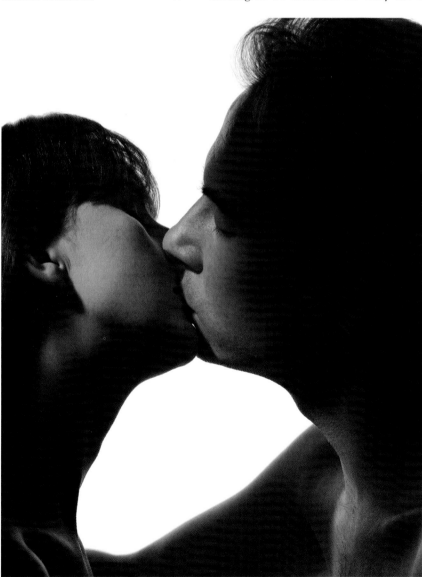

You must think of fantasies as nothing more than an elaborate daydream – and when of a sexual nature, certainly nothing to be ashamed of. They are a sign of a healthy and fertile imagination. And here's even better news: they are not even necessarily a sign of an unfulfilled sex life or relationship. On the contrary, there's every indication that those who have the most developed fantasies also have the most satisfying and loving relationships, the most active libidos and the most athletic bedtimes. Why do you think popular fantasies include sexy harems, being ravished by anonymous bodies and being watched while making love?

Yet most people are ashamed of their sexual daydreams and would never dream of discussing them – even with their spouse or partner. This is a pity, because the living out of fantasies can bring new and enormously fulfilling dimensions to any relationship.

What you must always remember is that you are no different to lovers all around the world. Fantasising is not being unfaithful to your partner. It is the opposite – it is wanting to please him or her while being pleasured yourself. Armed with that knowledge, you can begin to explore with your partner the areas where the fantasies overlap. You may realise there have been many missed moments when you and your partner have been enjoying similar fantasies in bed yet never realised it! What a waste! And just think of the heightened pleasure you can both have helping each other to 'play out' those fantasies you have kept secret all this time!

OPPOSITE: Fantasy sex should be fantastic fun for both of you.

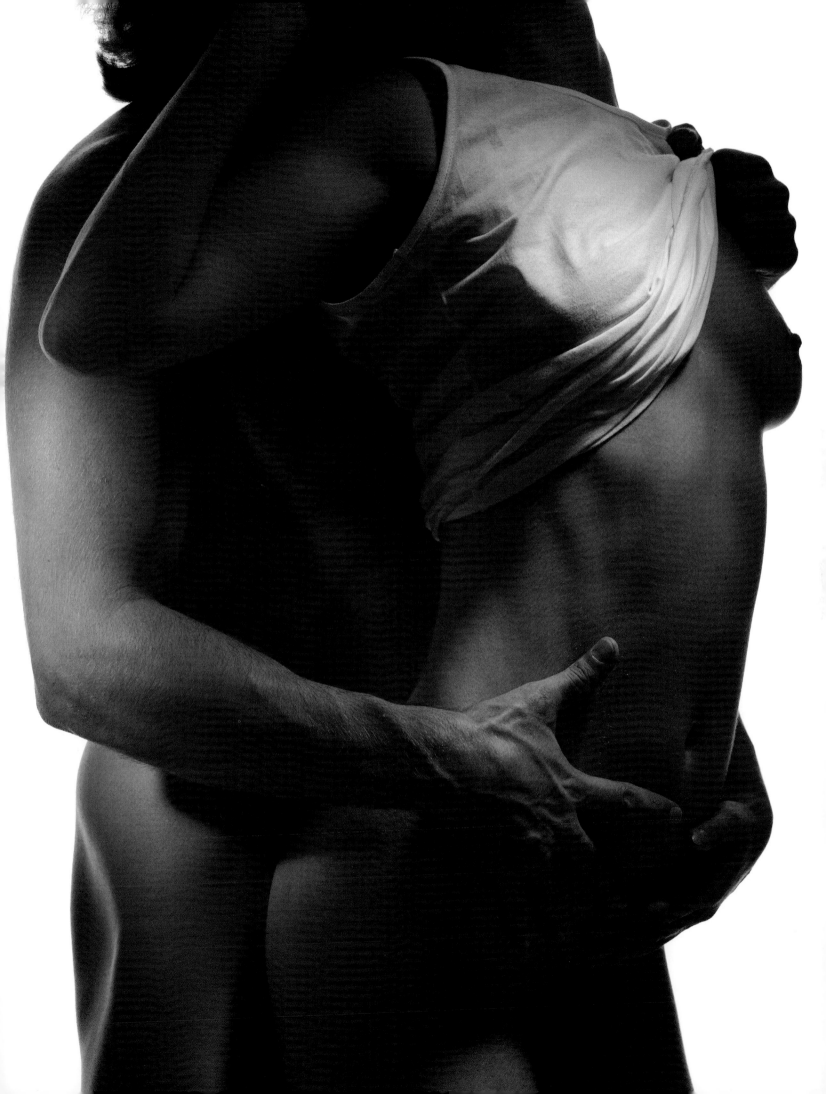

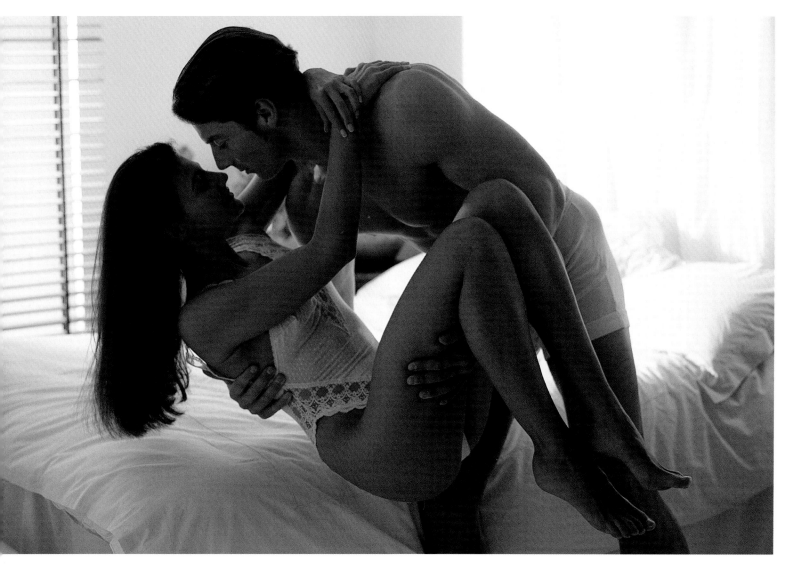

It is useful – and fun – to have a run-through of your sexual fantasy before approaching your partner with it. Have a defined beginning, middle and end as you create the sexy goings-on in your head. Make pictures come to mind, actually see and feel yourself in the centre of it all and experience the physical responses.

Having a 'practice run' like this guarantees that the fantasy actually works for you. If you get really aroused, it's a good fantasy for you. If you climax, you have created your very own Oscar-winning screenplay! You can also 'play' your fantasy through when your partner is making love to you. It will greatly enhance sexual activity or get you in the mood if you are not feeling particularly sexy.

You then need to decide if this is a fantasy you want to share with your partner. Lovers can feel inadequate if they believe their partner reaches an explosive orgasm only while thinking of their film idol or a band of randy sheikhs. There may be some fantasies you want to keep to yourself – but many others that will be bettered by sharing. And sharing all matters sexual is the ideal for a frank, fun and fulfilling relationship.

Like all sexual pleasure, fantasies are a learning experience. You just need the courage to talk about what fantasies really turn you on, that's why ideally you should read this book with your partner and be sensitive to what seems to excite them. Then is the time for some talking, some give and take, and negotiation.

Have fun. But remember, it's always wrong to force your partner – either physically or through emotional blackmail – to do anything he or she doesn't want to do. Fantasy sex should be fantastic fun for both of you.

The Four Types of Fantasy

The best research suggests that most fantasies fall into one of four main types: intimate, exploratory, impersonal or sado-masochistic.

'Intimate' fantasies are the most tame. They usually involve imagining that you're making love to your regular partner – perhaps in some exotic location, but possibly in your own bed.

'Exploratory' fantasies go beyond your ordinary sex life. Perhaps you bring in a third person or swap partners, get into an orgy or try out sex with someone of the same sex.

'Impersonal' fantasies don't feature other personalities. Maybe you have sex with someone else, but you don't regard them as a person. Or maybe you get off on blue movies, or dildos or rubber or dressing-up.

Finally, 'Sado-masochistic' fantasies are all about power within sex. They may involve bondage or spanking. In practice, most of these sado-masochistic fantasies are based around role-playing rather than inflicting pain, but they can still be very exciting.

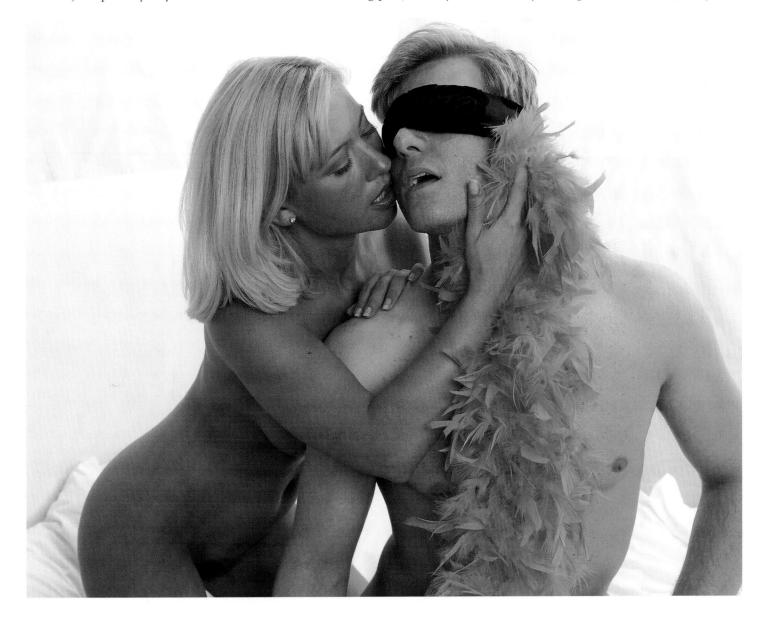

BELOW: Imagining making love with someone famous is a common fantasy.

OPPOSITE: Play out
the fantasies you have
kept secret all this time!

This part of the book is in four sections, each of which deals with one of these types of fantasy. So read all four. You may think that one of them is too tame or too racy now... but it would be a shame to miss out on the chance to acquire a whole new dream for yourself.

Intimate Fantasies

In this section we look at Intimate Fantasies. These make up the 'tamest' category and are usually daydreams about sex with your regular partner. Sometimes, of course, people add interesting twists. It might be imagining your partner dressed in a particular way, or playing out some role, or using a technique that you haven't tried in real life.

One of the most common of these twists is changing the location of love-making. If you

always have sex in bed, maybe you imagine it on the kitchen table, over the boss's desk at work or in a hotel lift.

But the most popular location shift is into the great outdoors. There are lots of reasons why making love in the open is such a popular fantasy. There's an amazing sense of freedom in being naked in the fresh air – just ask naturists! There are the new and exciting sensations of the cool earth and the fragrant grass hard against your writhing body. But above all there's that most delicious risk of being caught in the act!

Often the fantasy of outdoor love-making is more erotic than the reality. Certainly, ants' nests and sundry creepy-crawlies have been known to bring open-air sex sessions to a premature conclusion.

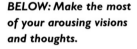

BELOW: Make the most
of your arousing visions
and thoughts.

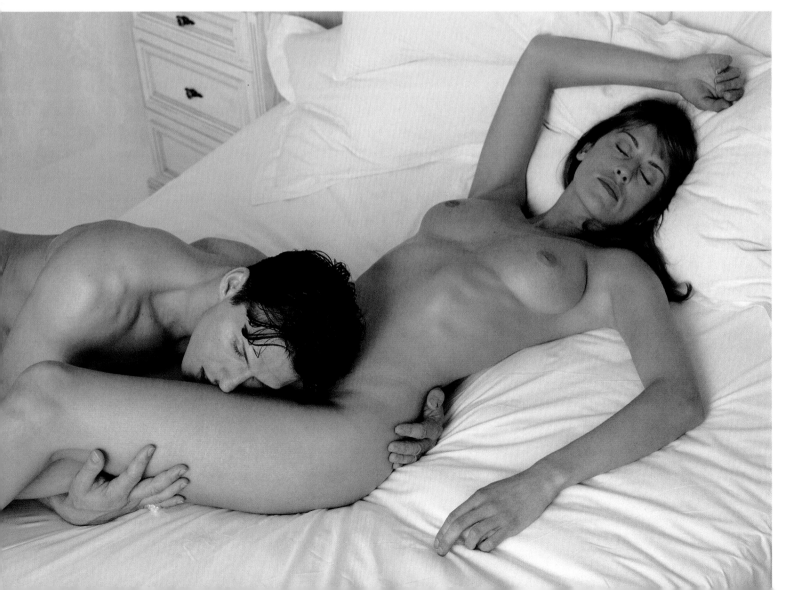

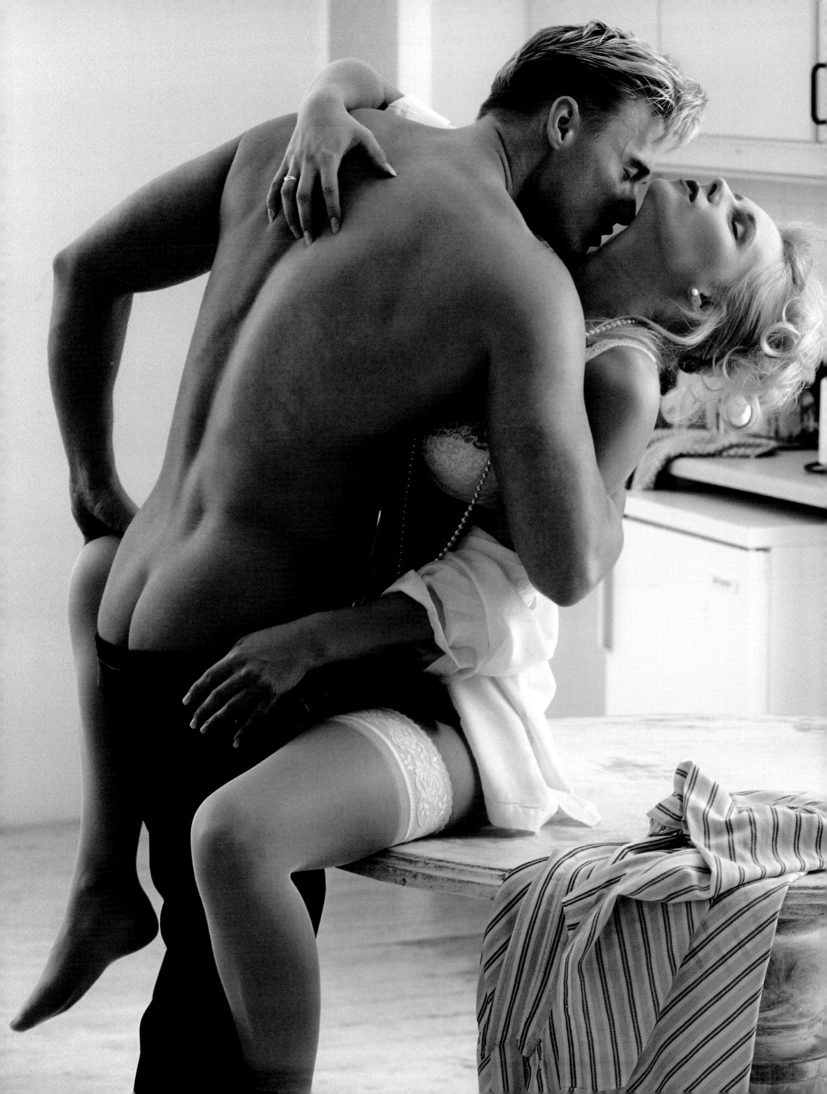

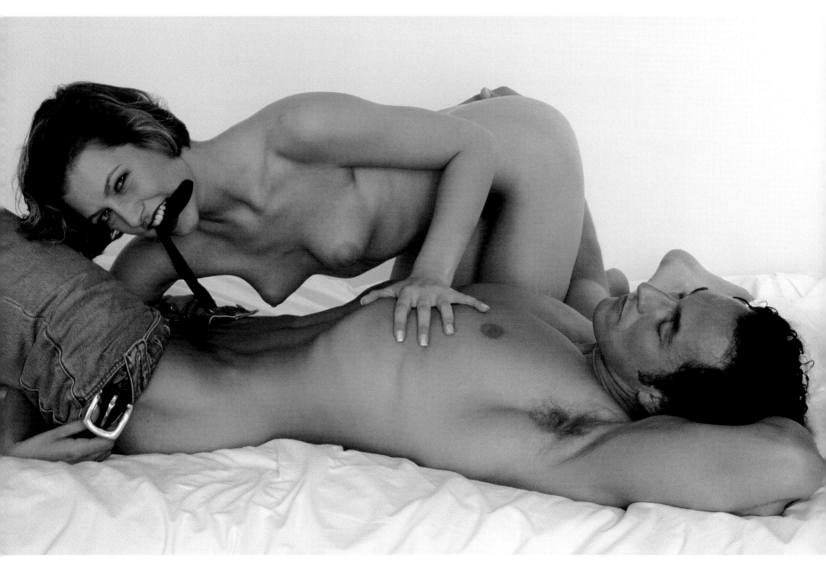

ABOVE: Come up with your very own Oscar-winning screenplay... including the climax!

A safer and altogether more comfortable variation on the 'change of location' theme is the romantic venue. In a fantasy, this is only limited by your imagination. If you want to act it out, it's limited by your budget.

Imagine making love to your partner in the master bedroom of a French chateau. Or in a penthouse roof garden, 40 floors above the streets of New York. Or in the plush, silky splendour of a Bedouin sheikh's tent.

You can place yourself in any location you please. Don't be constrained by your usual love-making techniques. As you fantasise, let your mind roam free to explore new possibilities, new positions and new sensations.

The fantasy of changing the location of your love-making is one way of breaking your sexual routine and so adding excitement. But it's by no means the only one.

Changing how you and your partner make love is equally exciting. Most people assume that this means varying your sexual repertoire – in other words, having a long 'menu' of techniques and picking different ones each time you have sex. Certainly, this helps to keep your sex life fresh and interesting, as does adding new techniques. But paradoxically, you can also get a great deal of sexual tension and enjoyment out of restricting what you practise in any one session.

The practice of self-restraint and self-discipline can be remarkably rewarding. Try agreeing in advance that you *won't* do what you normally do.

Let's assume that usually you enjoy extensive foreplay, including oral sex, as you lead up to full sexual intercourse. But on this occasion you should decide to restrict yourselves to mutual masturbation. As you fight off you impulses to escalate your activity, you will find that you are exquisitely teasing yourself and your partner other. The orgasm that can be achieved by that sort of mutual teasing is often more intense than the ones you get from routine 'full' sex. Variations on this fantasy include keeping on some clothing or even stimulating each other when fully clothed. The latter needs some rougher handling than normal, and both are made more fun if you and your partner use your mouths.

Oral fantasies can fit into the self-restraint fantasy, if oral sex is normally a part of your routine love-making, or into a whole fantasy in its own right if it's something you have never done with your partner. Oral sex has never been so popular, but it's still quite rare among some population groups, and for them it's one of the most common fantasies.

When we speak, our mouths are uniquely capable of communicating pleasure to our loved ones. The same applies when we make love. The use of the mouth when kissing mouth to mouth, when kissing and licking other parts of your partner's body and when stimulating your partner's genitals is one of the tenderest, most loving and most giving acts.

Whether as a self-restraint fantasy or simply as a daydream by which we excite ourselves, oral sex is probably the ultimate favourite. That's hardly surprising: to be on the receiving end of a skilfully manipulating tongue is to experience one of the world's most sensual experiences.

BELOW: Use your mouth to bring you and your partner together in mutual, sexual bliss.

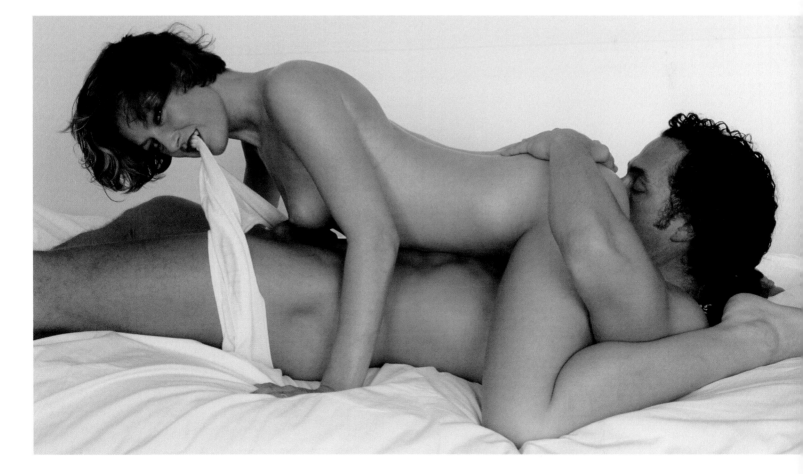

OPPOSITE: For some the reality of carrying out a fantasy threesome is a highly exciting possibility.

BELOW: Exploratory fantasies need not involve the physical presence of a third person, and thus remain an imaginary act.

Exploratory Fantasies

The fantasies we have looked at so far are the easiest to put into effect, in that they are, at most, mild extensions to your existing sex life. Daydreams in the next category, 'Exploratory Fantasies', are also very common, but they are more difficult to live out because they involve at least one person beyond your regular partner.

Faithfulness is still very much at a premium in most relationships. With the threat of AIDS, it's perhaps more valued than ever. That means that it's often difficult for a person in a long-term relationship to bring up the subject of fantasies involving others. If you are thinking of raising the topic with your partner, think about it carefully – some people would rather end a relationship than contemplate the thought of 'sharing' their loved one with a third party. And while many may find the idea of bringing in a neighbour or dinner guest to share a fantasy threesome highly exciting, many might be made to feel that they are simply not enough to keep their partner satisfied.

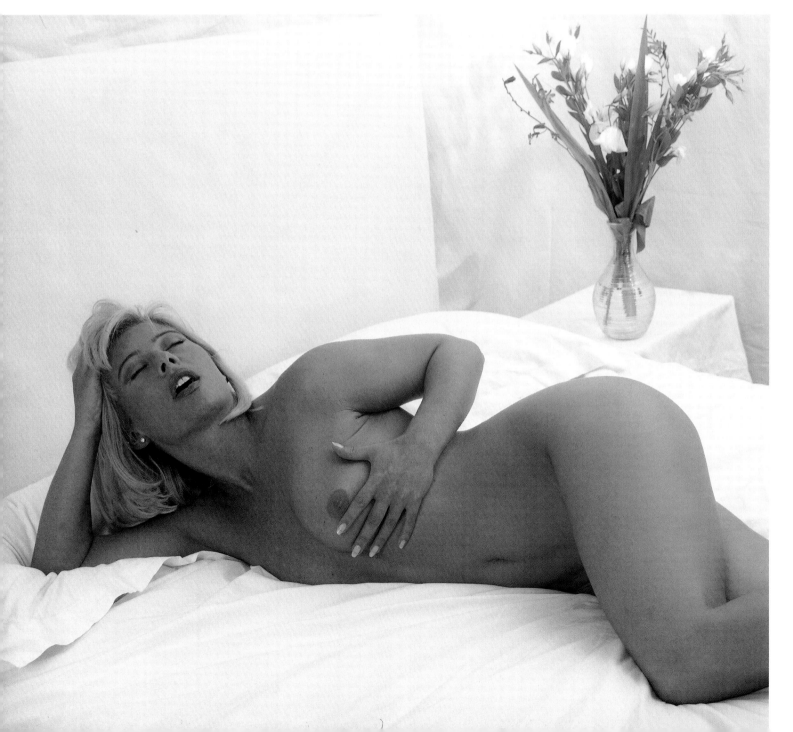

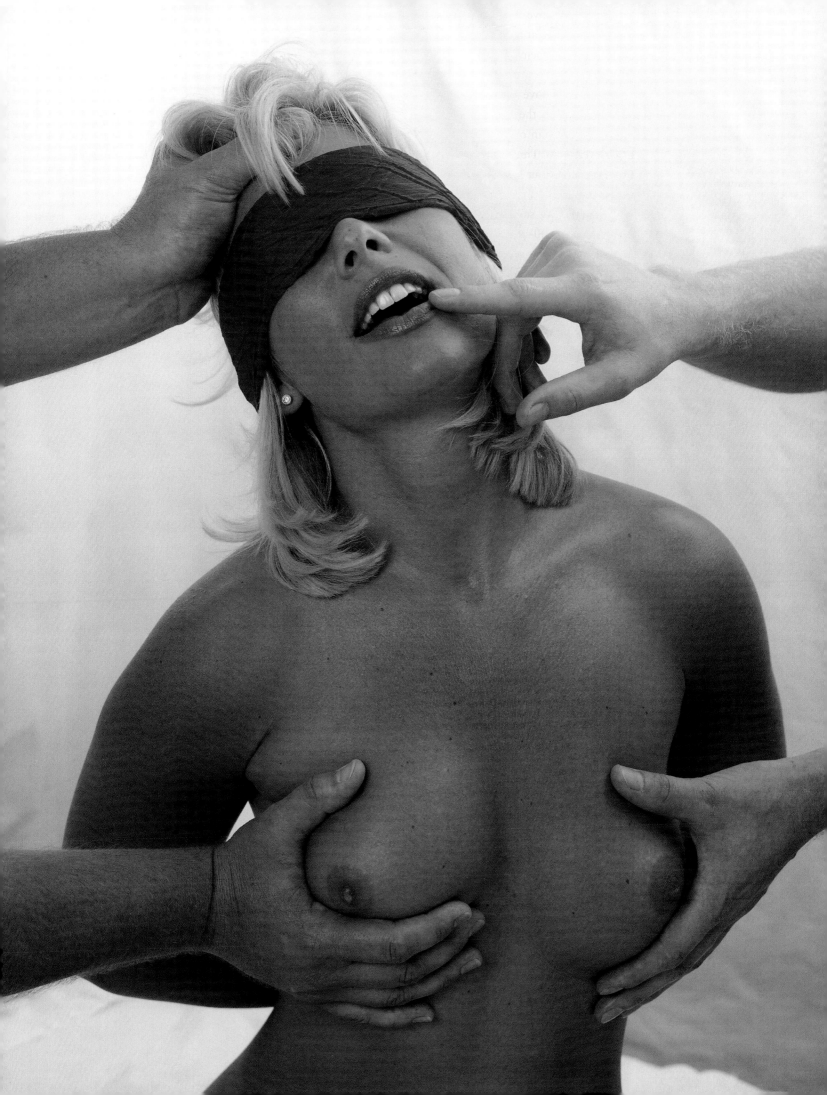

Exploratory fantasies are much more common in men than women, and there may be some truth in the idea that men are naturally the more promiscuous. But of course, there are exceptions. A significant number of women fantasise about having sex with a number of different men. This can take the form of serial promiscuity (where the woman has a string of separate sexual encounters) or group promiscuity (where the woman is serviced by a number of men within the same encounter). Sometimes the woman may take on two or more men at the same moment. For example, she may engage in sexual intercourse with one man while performing oral sex on another.

Men's group fantasies are similar, revolving around pleasuring several women in one sex session. Men, traditionally encouraged to believe that 'many makes you much more macho', are aroused by the idea of having sex with more than one woman at a time. And what better way to prove to himself that he's more than capable of

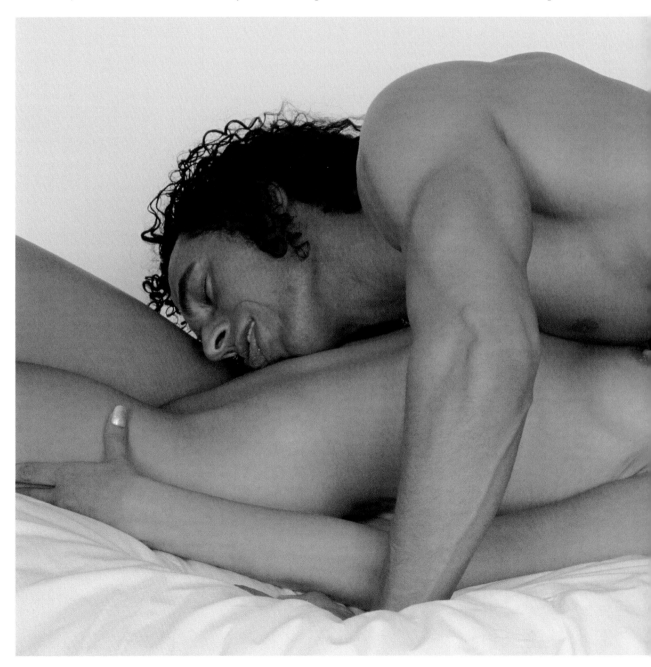

RIGHT: You must summon up the courage to talk to your partner about which fantasies really turn you on.

performing well for one woman when in his dreams he can leave a whole bed-full exhausted and satisfied!

For both sexes, such fantasies highlight the need to be seen as sexy and attractive without any threat of jealousy or breakdown of a relationship – and what's wrong with that?

Fantasising about sex with a stranger is straightforward. It's simple sex without having to shake hands and introduce yourselves! In other words, no niceties are involved and there's no need to meet again. You have a steamy sex session that's unforgettable.

Sex-with-a-stranger fantasies are probably the most simple to understand because they are about simple sex! You can walk away with no guilt and it has not been necessary to reveal anything about yourself. And, unlike the harsh reality, there is no threat of contacting a sexual disease, discovering an unwanted pregnancy or sexual play turning nasty and spiralling out of your control. You are controlling the stranger's behaviour towards you.

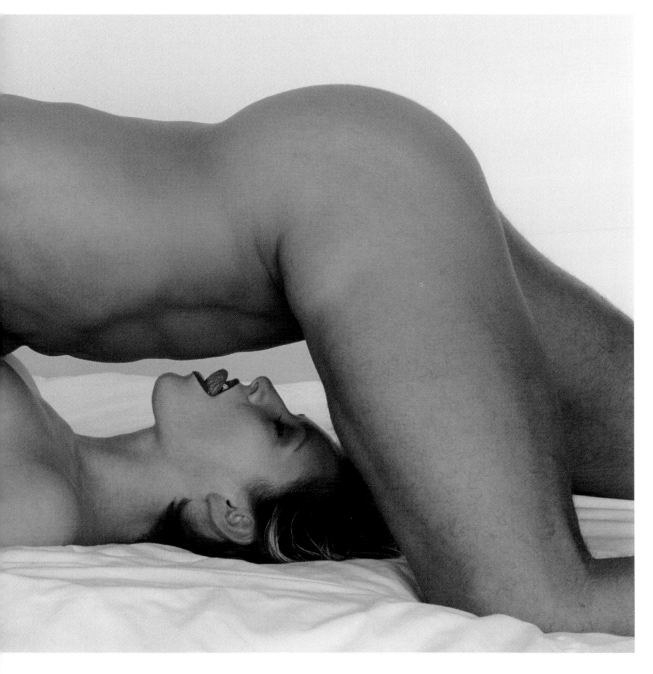

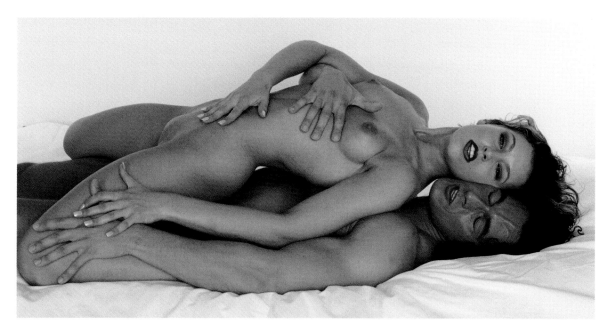

It is no wonder that many women's stranger fantasies feature everyone from a carpet-fitter to a builder, complete with hard-hat! And what better way to enjoy no-holds-barred sex with not an ounce of guilt than to 'become' a prostitute.

When it comes to fantasising about sex with someone of the same sex, it should make you feel more comfortable to know that this doesn't mean your own sexuality is in any doubt. Indeed, such fantasies can actually bring you more in touch with your sexual needs.

Impersonal Fantasies

Sex toys, porn films and 'headless' partners all play their part in impersonal fantasies. It's like having sex without the hassle of having a partner! But what can you do with a sex toy or blue movie in a fantasy that you can't do for real, you may ask. This is where your imagination runs riot.

Some men and women fantasise about using giant-size dildos in their sex-play – or having a stranger 'inflict' pleasure on them with a bizarre sex toy. Incredible sex items are dreamed up by some people, involving everything from highly advanced laboratory experiments to the most amazing sexually-gratifying equipment, on which the fantasiser reclines in front of a roomful of observers! As noted earlier, the imagination of real people far exceeds that of fictional characters!

As with all fantasies, exploratory ones mean you are free to enjoy pleasure that the 'real you' would be afraid to admit. Just who is doing what to who doesn't matter in these fantasies, it's what is being used that becomes the focus.

The movies that flicker across your own secret 'screen' have you as director – meaning you can create weird and wonderful sexual situations hotter than anything than can be bought. You may even be the 'star' of the film but, because it's not the real you, the whole fantasy becomes impersonal – a sexy image that arouses the real you. Again, this sort of fantasy means you can engage in sexual activities that would be unlikely, even undesirable, in everyday life.

The important thing is to make the most of these arousing visions and thoughts. Do not feel guilty if the images in your head are far removed from what you would normally do and do not involve your regular partner. Use your arousal to bring you and your partner together in mutual, sexual bliss.

'Headless' or 'unseen partners' feature in the fantasies of those who feel guilty about being sexually alluring. These fantasies are more likely to be enjoyed by women than men – although occasionally a man gets turned on by the idea of an anonymous woman doing all sorts of sexual things to him without being asked. The female fantasiser doesn't need to worry about who is pleasuring her, concentrating purely on the effect of her faceless lover and ensuring he does exactly what she wants him to do. Such fantasies can be taken one step further by the fantasiser whispering his or her thoughts and images, or by getting their partner to play along, talking dirty and sharing the fantasy.

As with every aspect of sex in this book, get the most fun you can from your fantasies and make your most secret sexy stories regular bedtime 'reading'.

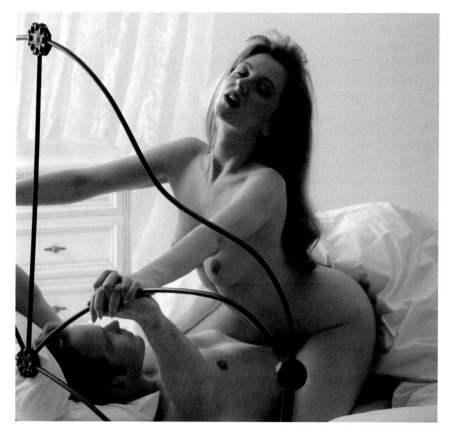

Sado-Masochistic Fantasies

These are all about pain and power that would be dangerous to play out for real. In simple terms, sadism involves gaining sexual pleasure or orgasm by inflicting pain on another; masochism is when the recipient of pain becomes sexually aroused.

It may be shocking that some women fantasise about being taken by force – in what really constitutes rape – but the crucial difference from reality is that the woman enjoys what is happening to her. She is in control the whole time and enjoys the feeling of sexual pleasure 'against her will'. That's why being tied-up and unable to prevent yourself being pleasured is a favourite fantasy for women (and popular pastime for real, too!). Bondage is a very common fantasy, with the woman closing her eyes and imagining herself being gently tied to a four-poster and the man fantasising he's doing the tying!

ABOVE: Pick a different technique from your 'menu' each time you have sex.

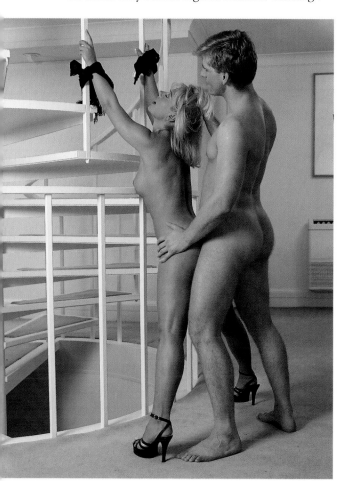

LEFT: Tied up and pleasured "against her will" is a popular fantasy for a lot of women.

It is not surprising to learn that the majority of female sexual fantasies are passive, with the man doing all the hard work. Some men say they want to tie down their partner for sex so that she will have to accept her own sexuality. For though women won't always admit it, they can get very aroused when made to have sex while tied down because of this forced acceptance.

This applies, too, to fantasies involving sexual humiliation – but great sexual satisfaction. For men this could be domination by a woman or women who inflict pain. Many men enjoy being beaten on command, verbally abused and treated in a demeaning way. For them, being 'punished' is ideal foreplay for explosive sex.

Sado-masochism fantasies certainly prove how close pain is linked to pleasure! But it's not just men who like being hurt. Women can enjoy having their bottoms smacked just as much and pretend to cry for mercy. And sometimes just the

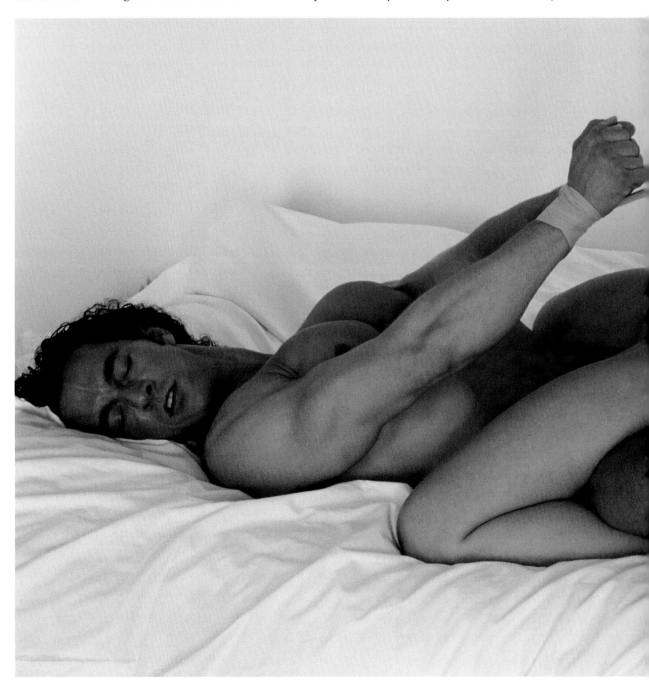

anticipation of the touch of a whip or the back of a hand is enough to sexually arouse them.

Most of these sado-masochistic fantasies involve enforced, guilt-free submission to a world of sexual abandonment and wild fun. So it is natural that fear plays a part in these sorts of fantasies, too. Who can blame you for 'giving in' to the most outrageous and perverted demands (which you secretly enjoy to frenzied heights, of course) when you are frightened for your very life!

Such fantasies mean you can masturbate without bad feelings – who can refuse when a terrifying intruder is holding a knife to your throat? – and reach delicious orgasm without guilt. It is no wonder that the French call orgasm 'le petit mort' – little death – as many sex experts believe that sex and the fear of death are closely linked!

BELOW: Open your mind to new experiences.

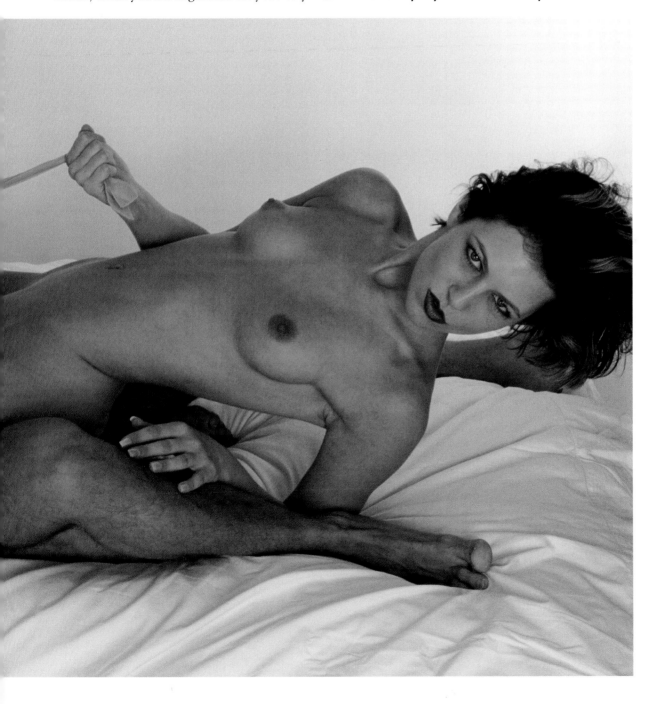

5 FULFILMENT

How do you ensure you enjoy a fine sex finale? The answer is simple: Have fun sex! Laughing and loving, as we have shown, are parallel paths in a perfect physical relationship. They are the prelude to a great climax. But some people still find that breakthrough difficult – or impossible. Men don't seem to have as much trouble as women in this direction! A surprising number of women still think it's wrong to let on that the experience of love-making is pleasurable. There are women who think men should do all the work, and who barely move during intercourse! This chapter demonstrates the importance of movement and position in achieving the most perfect orgasms. We imagine the different positions that allow both partners to move in different ways and be in total control of the proceedings when it comes to speed, rhythm and technique.

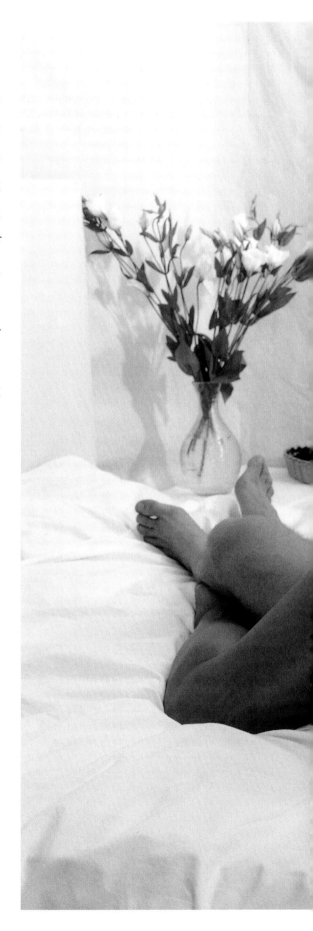

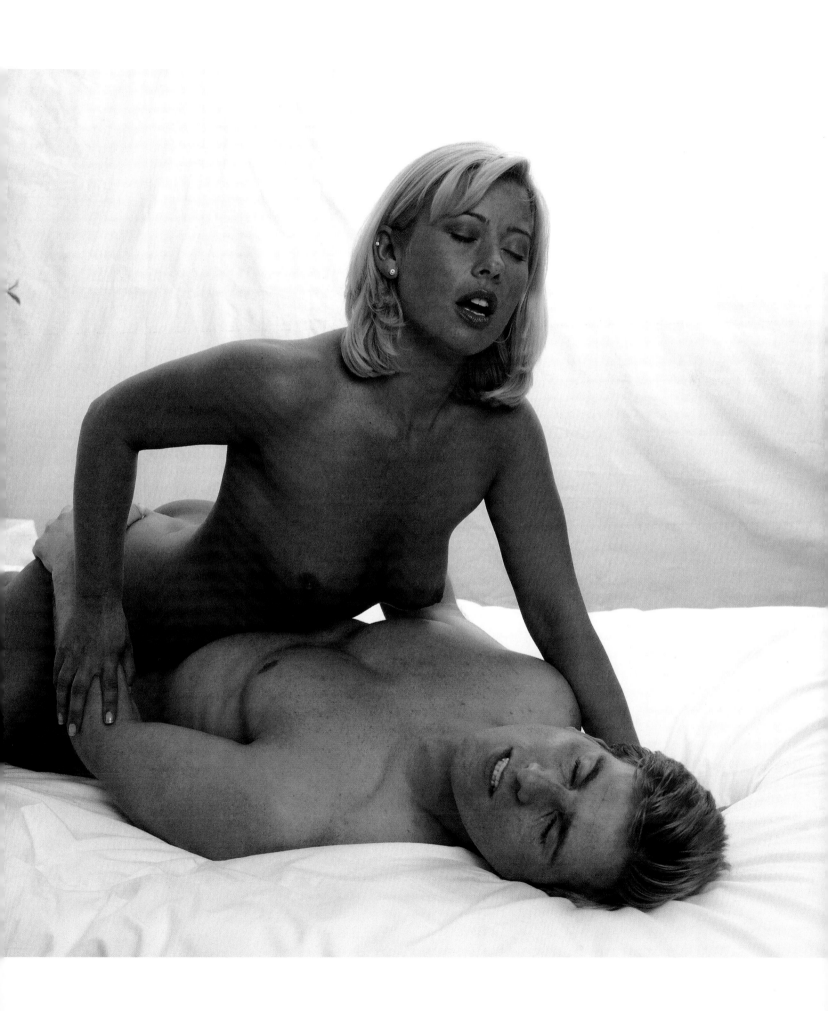

Hopefully, by now you have learned that laughing and loving should be a regular part of sex. After all, the object of this book is to bring FUN back to the physical side of your relationship.

That's all well and good, you may ask, but how can we guarantee a great climax as well as a great chuckle?! Ideally, of course, making love results in both of you reaching total sexual satisfaction. And that's what this chapter is all about – finding out that fun and fulfilment go blissfully together when it comes to making love.

Looking for fulfilment can be just as much fun as finding it. We're not talking about having as many sexual partners as possible – that's not fun, it's farcical. (Indiscriminate sex should also carry a health warning.) No, what we want is a lovely, comfortable and sexy journey into the unknown with the partner who means a lot to you.

Arriving at a joyful state of satisfaction could take time, however. For instance, did you know that the vast majority of couples make love at 10pm on Fridays? Isn't that a bit like setting your video recorder?

Make a decision to make love the moment you wake up. Who could resist the arousing alarm clock of gentle, sleepy kisses and caresses all over the body? Or go to bed earlier and spend *all* the time *until* 10pm having sex. Or why go to bed at all? How about halfway up the stairs or in the bath? For the really loving and adventurous couple, there are no restrictions on the where and when. Find different times, locations and ways of making love. After reading previous chapters you should now be brave enough to talk about what turns you on.

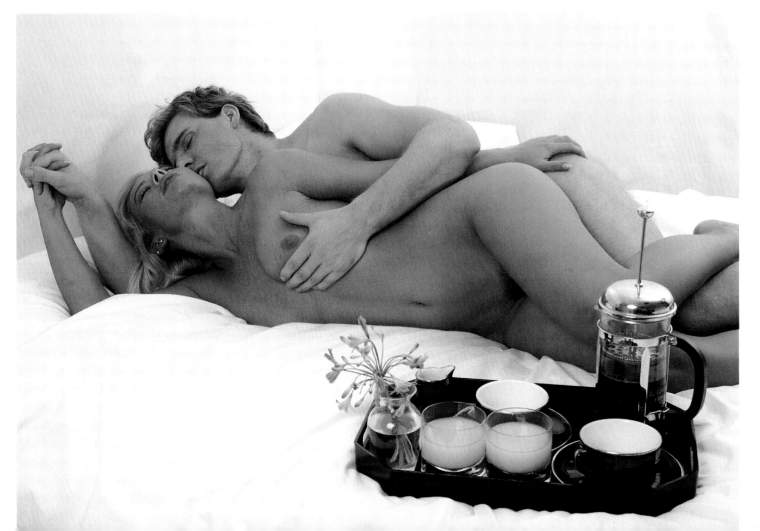

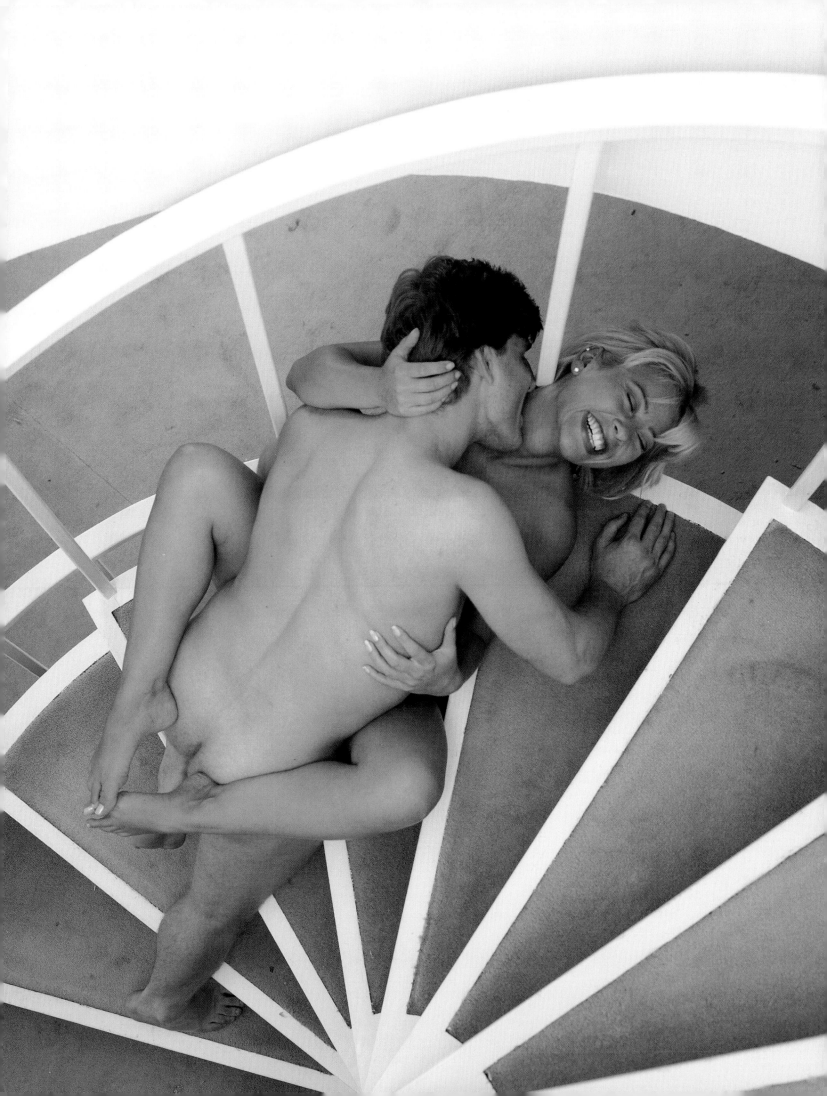

Your imagination should come into play. If you want a totally fulfilled sex life, think for yourself of ways to brighten it – and express those thoughts. There's one word which will set you off on to the road of mutually fantastic sex and that's 'experiment'. Want to ensure that, even if the relationship eventually fails because of other factors, you and your new partner have a great time in bed? Experiment. Want to break the boredom of routine sex in a long-established partnership? Experiment.

It could simply be making love in a different way or acting out a favourite fantasy. Never be afraid to try something new – though as has been emphasised throughout *Fun Sex*, *both* of you should find it fun. Why not start with some or all of the following....

Ten Positions to Tickle Your Fancy

Sleepy Sex

Minimum effort, maximum pleasure. The man lies on his side and the woman lies with her back to him. Her legs go over his side and her bottom nestles against his penis so that he can enter her from the rear. She either rocks him back and forth or moves herself backwards and forwards with her legs. This position is good for pregnant women or if one of you has a back problem.

Top-to-Toe Titillation

Or sex in a stretch! The woman starts by sitting on top of the man with his penis inside her. She then stretches out on top of him, head-to-head and toe-to-toe. Instead of riding up and down, she moves forwards and backwards, stimulating her clitoris against his penis. It's great for women who enjoy their clitoris getting attention during intercourse.

Puppy Love

Brings out animal instincts. The woman kneels on all fours and the man enters her from behind. It's real nickname is 'doggy fashion', which puts some people off. Others find the idea of 'mating' like animals particularly exciting – it's a position where the woman feels very much 'taken' by the dominant male. Variations include the woman lying on her stomach or kneeling over a chair, bed, pillow, table – anything that's the right height. This position allows the man to caress the woman's breasts and clitoris to ensure orgasm is reached.

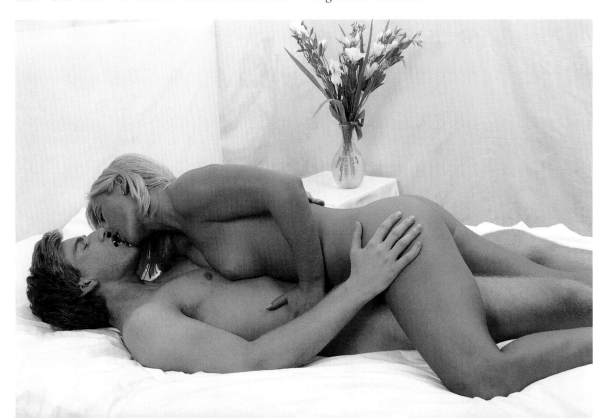

RIGHT: Stretch out for
top-to-toe titillation.

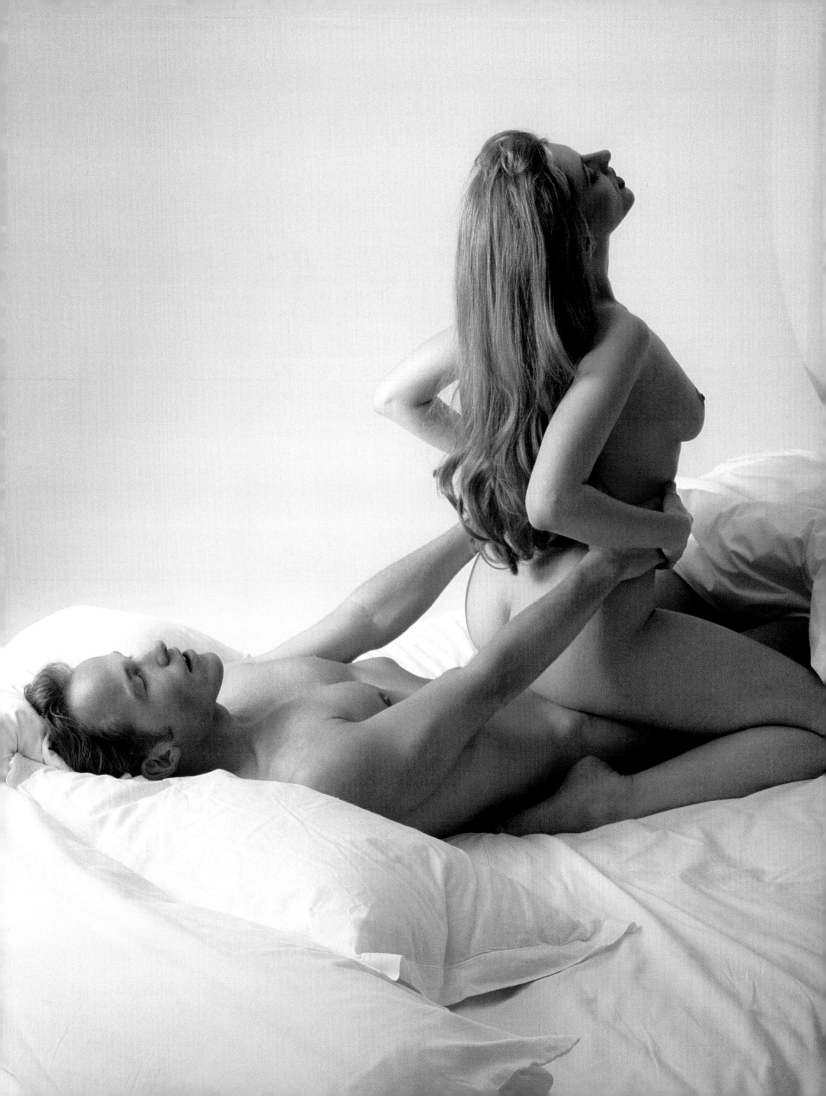

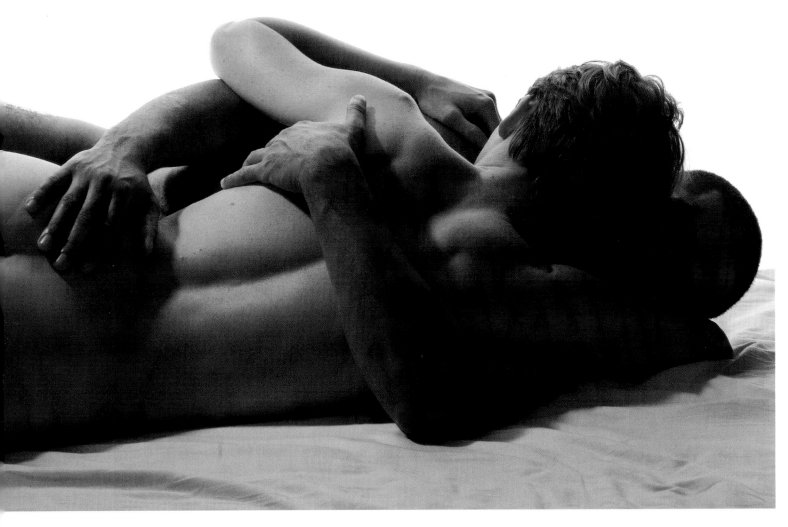

ABOVE: Spice up your sex life with a variety of new sexual positions.

Sexy Spoons

Snugly sex. The woman and man lie on their sides, the man behind the woman – just like two spoons in your cutlery draw! Again, the man enters from the rear. Another position that's comfortable if the woman is pregnant.

Girls on Top

For the woman who likes to take charge. The man lies on his back and the woman lies on top. Her legs can be either astride or between his. This is an ideal position for a pregnant woman because there is so little pressure on the abdomen. Men particularly like this position because the woman has her hands free to caress him and guide his hands. He, too, is in a very much 'hands-on' position and will find the going less tiring.

The Chair

Your man is a lovely, sexy cushion. He sits in a chair and the woman sits on his lap, facing away from him. He enters her from below. A variation is for the woman to sit sideways across his lap or facing him, which allows the man to pay more attention with his tongue or hands to her breasts.

Stand and Deliver

Enough to make anyone walk tall. But this position is helped if the two of you aren't wildly different heights – if this is the case, a stool is very useful! The man stands up and the woman wraps her legs around his thighs while he supports her. This is a good position to play in the shower or even the sea (as long as no one's looking).

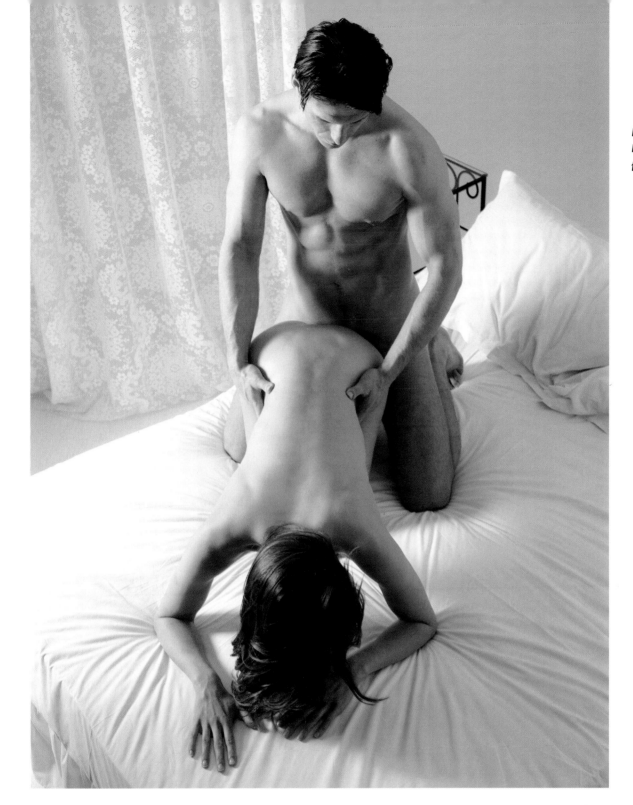

LEFT: Rear entry can be thrilling for both partners.

Nice 'n' Kneesy

This is no mean feat, either. The woman lies on her back with her knees up and her feet flat on the bed. The man supports his weight on his hands and enters her from above.

Feet First

You need to be fit for this one. The woman adopts the same position as 'Nice 'n' Kneesy', but this time puts her ankles over the man's shoulders.

Right Angles

Or a bit on the side! The woman lies on her back, legs drawn up, feet flat on the bed or held up by grasping behind the knees. The man is on his side at right angles to her body as he enters her. This is an excellent position for helping a woman have an orgasm as it enables the man to caress her clitoris and breasts easily while inside her.

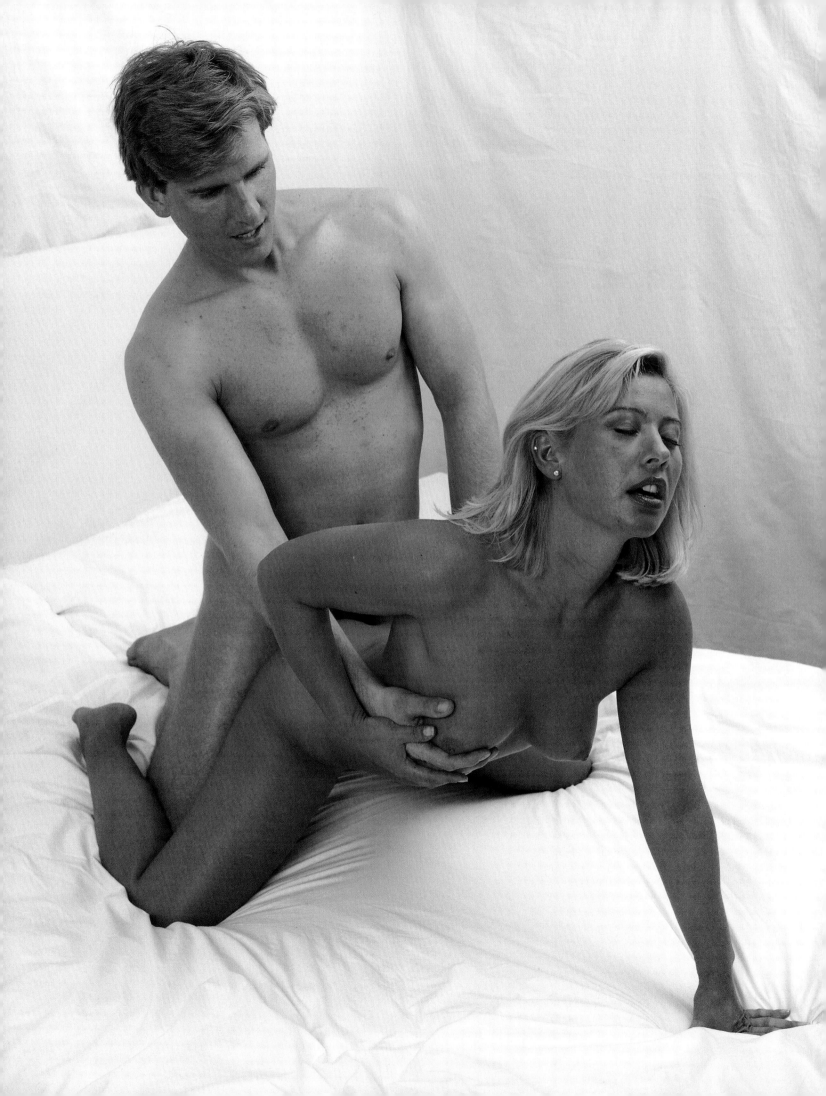

It's probably stating the obvious, but all love-making requires some movement. (Though you would surprised at the number of women who still think it's wrong to let on the experience is pleasant and dare not move! There are also women who think men should do all the work.) Different positions mean both of you can move in different ways. In general, the one on top is in control of the proceedings when it comes to speed, rhythm and technique. On the whole, men prefer positions which provide deeper penetration and women enjoy positions which give some of their outer bits stimulation.

While we're on this subject, the existence of the woman's G-spot has been the cause of much discussion. Some insist they haven't got one. Some men can't be bothered to look for it. But the G-spot lies in the lower third of the front wall of a woman's vagina. It can best be stimulated in love-making positions from behind, where the man can angle his penis to hit the right spot.

OPPOSITE: Hitting the G-spot: this is best stimulated with the man positioned behind.

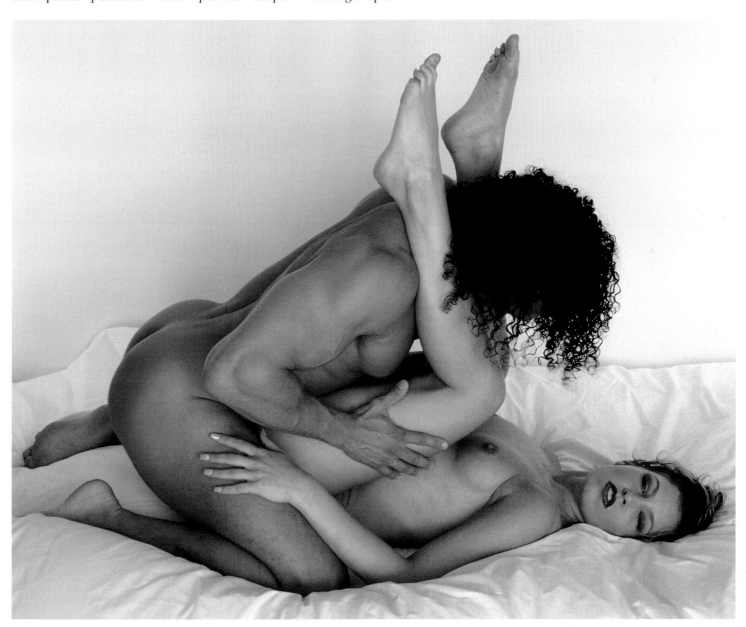

ABOVE: Experiment... and set yourself on the road to mutually great sex.

Love-Making Mechanics

We don't always understand how some of nature's most beautiful creations work, we just know that we love the result. How exactly does a flower's petals emerge into such splendid colour, for instance? Why do butterflies start life as caterpillars?

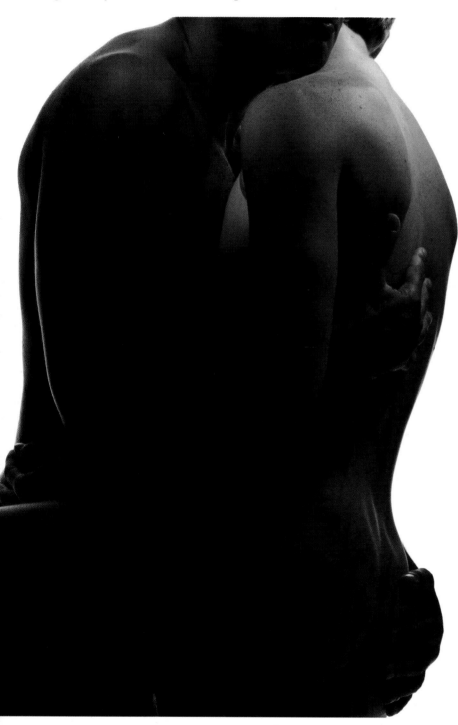

Another question you're probably asking is why have we diverged from the subject of sex. Well, I'm trying to make the point that while you can go through life in ignorant bliss of many wonderful occurrences around you, there is one truly exquisite thing you *should* understand the mechanics of, and that is the workings of the male and female body during love-making.

For many, it is all a mystery, but unless you at least know the basics of physical changes leading to orgasm, how can you possibly understand each other's bodies? And how can you give your partner an orgasm – the ultimate in sexual fulfilment? So for those who are happy enough to be taken back to school in such sexual matters (and for those who pretend they know it all), here is the *Fun Sex* guide to your body's machinery:

The Woman

As sexual excitement mounts, extra blood accumulates quickly in the genital area. This happens in both men and women and the technical name is vasocongestion. In women, this blood flow forces natural tissue fluid through the walls of the vagina, producing nature's very own lubricating oils. The nipples become erect, the dark area (areola) of the nipple becomes even darker and the breasts increase in size. Pulse rate and blood pressure rise. At this stage, a 'sex rash' usually appears, starting at the top of the stomach and spreading to the breasts.

Shortly before orgasm, the inner lips (labia) of the vagina turn a deeper red and the vagina lengthens and widens, with the clitoris retracting.
Hello Orgasm: The uterus and outer third of the vagina go into a series of fast contractions. The number varies greatly.
Bye-Bye Orgasm: The pulse, blood pressure and breathing rate return to normal. The labia loses its redness, the sex rash fades and the nipples are no longer erect. The vagina goes back to its normal size.

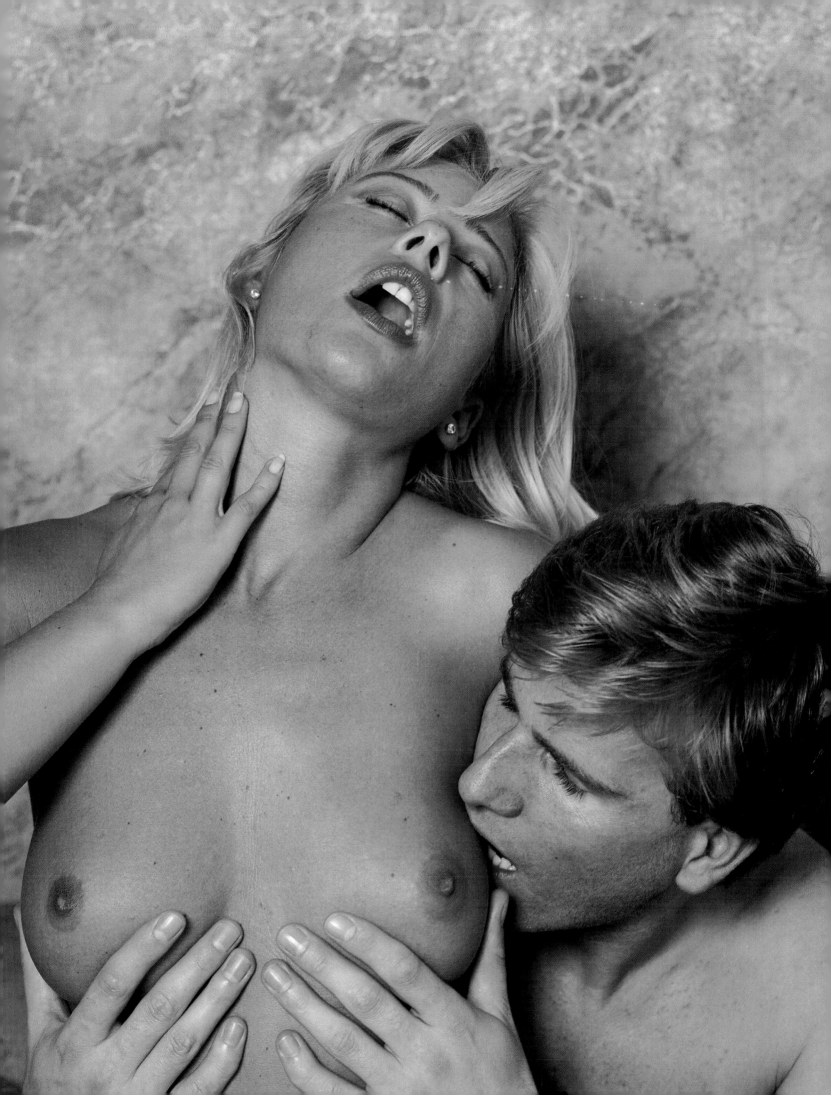

RIGHT: Often the man needs to exert great self-control to allow his partner to reach her climax.

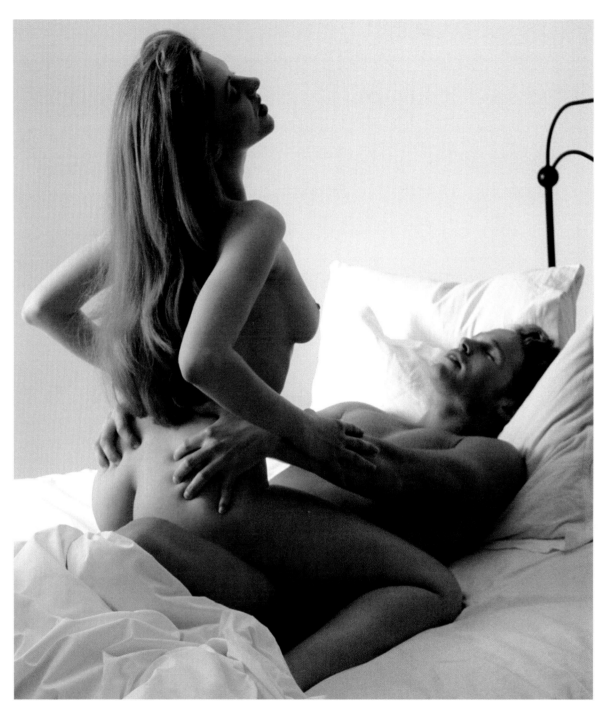

Come Again? For a woman to have more than one orgasm through sexual intercourse, the man has to exercise great self-control. This isn't easy – he has to provide good, strong, penetrative sex without having a climax himself. This should, however, give the woman her 'starter' orgasm – always the strongest of the lot.

A vibrator or masturbation are alternative ways to induce this first climax or could be used as nice little 'follow-ups'. In fact, many women can only have an orgasm through direct simulation of the clitoris – for them, penetrative sex doesn't hit the spot at all. However you go for the multiple orgasmic experience, you'll need a rest in between. Whatever those sexy novels say, the body cannot explode into one earth-shattering orgasm after another without having a breather.

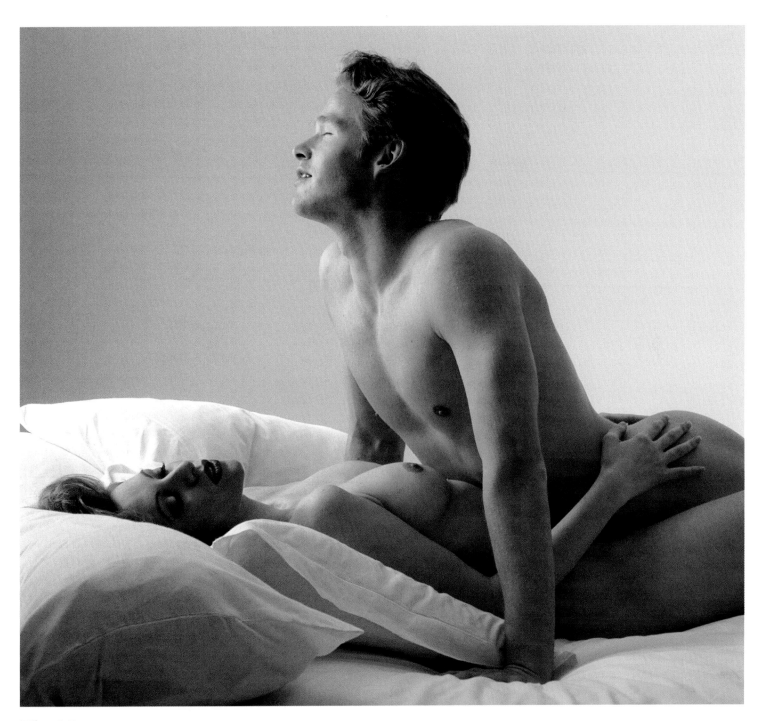

The Man

Vasocongestion in men is evident in an erection. It is caused by the blood flowing into the spongy tissue of the penis, causing it to swell. Both men and women experience an involuntary tensing of the muscles throughout the body. Pulse rate, blood pressure and breathing rate increases. Nipples become hard.

Some men have a sex flush similar to that a woman experiences.

Hello Orgasm: A man has two stages of orgasm. The first is the semen collecting at the entrance of the urethra – and from here there is no turning back! Contractions of the ejaculatory ducts and muscles around the penis in the second stage of orgasm then force the semen out.

ABOVE: Fun and fulfilment go blissfully together when it comes to making love.

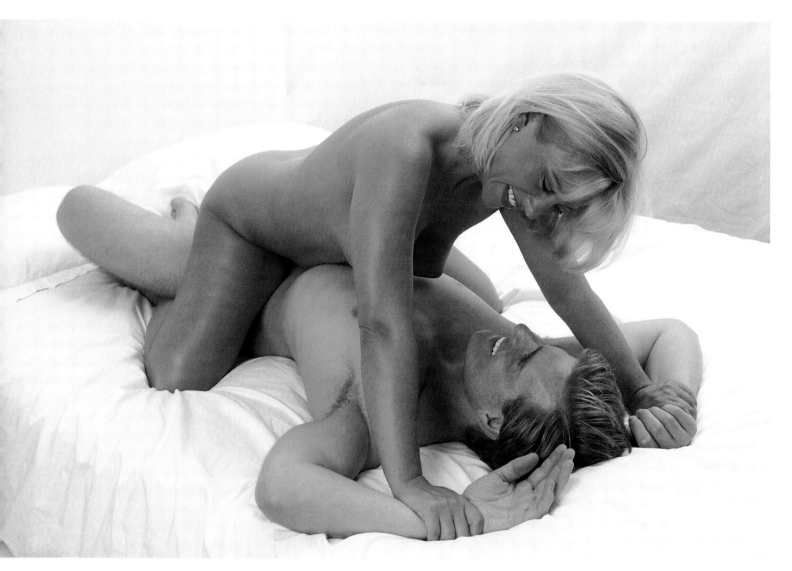

*ABOVE: It can be
highly arousing for
both partners when
the woman takes
the initiative.*

Bye-Bye Orgasm: The contractions subside, the erection goes and nipples soften.

Come Again? Again, don't believe those raunchy sex tales where the stud of a man has his woman begging for mercy with one giant, active erection after another. Though some men can keep an erection after their climax, an awful lot more simply won't respond, no matter what tantalising stimulation you offer. Some multi-orgasmic men ejaculate at the first go, some at the last and some in between. You can probably 'train' yourself to have more than one ejaculation in a single sex session by mastering the art of self-control. But just like other aspects of love-making, it is important to remember you are not trying to break any records.

A Few Factors of Fulfilling Sex

Communication – mental and physical: Talk about your fears, fantasies and funny ways. Ask what your partner likes, loves and lusts for. Show each other what touches you find titillating and a turn-on. Your partner should also be your best friend – and don't you tell your best friend *everything*?

He likes: you to get the ball rolling sometimes (men get fed up making the first move every time); excitement (men believe variety is the spice of a love life); being loved (yes, men have feelings, too).

She likes: you to give her plenty of time before full sex (women need longer than men to get in the mood physically and mentally, so long, lingering

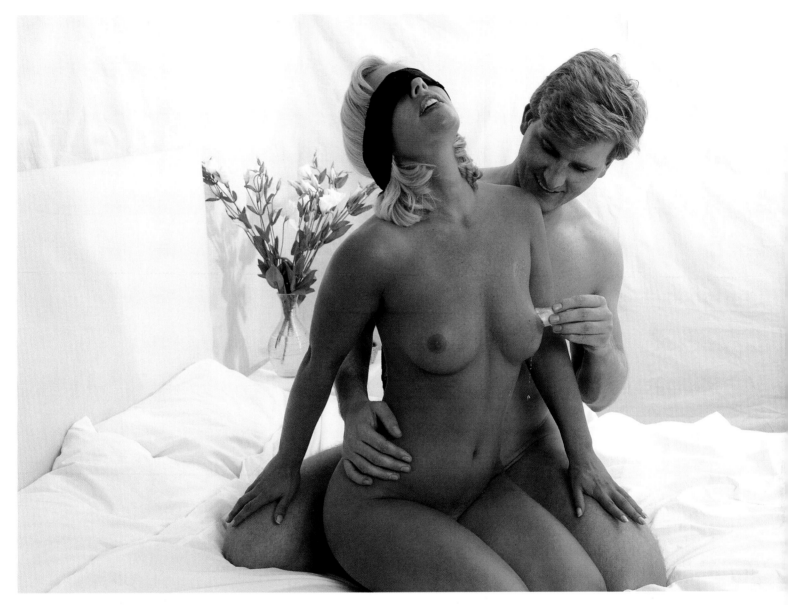

foreplay is crucial); tenderness (no woman likes to feel she's just a body to be used); understanding (there's no shortcut here – you *have* to learn those little touches mean a lot).

Sex is not a weapon: It should therefore NEVER be used in a threatening way or as the focus for anger, punishment or blackmail.

Love-making is not a race: Don't forget to pause for cuddles, kisses and caresses. Reaching a climax in as fast a time as possible is not the aim and slowing things down to savour the feel of skin on skin brings about a special feeling of closeness.

Will You Be a Sexy Sexagenarian?

There's probably one big question that you have been asking yourselves as you read through this book, and that is: 'Is it really possible to make love to the same person for the rest of your life?' An awful lot of people think so. And apart from helping books like this one to sell, it's a question that's answered by couples who actually *want* a long-term relationship to work.

If you see the 20, 30, 40 or even 60 years ahead of you as a nightmare instead of being full of dreams, perhaps your current relationship isn't for you. If you don't pay heed to aspects of your

ABOVE: Act out your fantasies to achieve prolonged and original foreplay.

relationship such as romance, consideration, pleasant surprises and understanding, how can you expect to have a brilliant time in bed? Your partner won't want to give their all to someone who gives so little. As one my favourite sexperts once said, 'You both have to work hard at relieving the monogamy!' That's worth bearing in mind when you consider that the average couple will make love more than 4,000 times if they stay together for life.

It won't all be plain sailing as you go through life together. For a start, it's important for men to understand their own sexual abilities and how they will change in later life. It's equally important for women to understand it. And vice-versa for

women. Ladies, you may not want to face the hard facts about getting older, but your body will face them for you, and your partner will have to appreciate this, too.

So here is a brief guide to ensure you both know what to expect from each other – and can tailor your sexual demands accordingly.

WOMEN: Sorry, but your man's most active sexual period was long before you ever got him into the bedroom. It was when he'd just reached puberty and his hormones were crying out to be noticed!

Those hormones start to drop slightly when he's in his 20s and after a few years most men stop

BELOW: Men sometimes enjoy their partner making the first move.

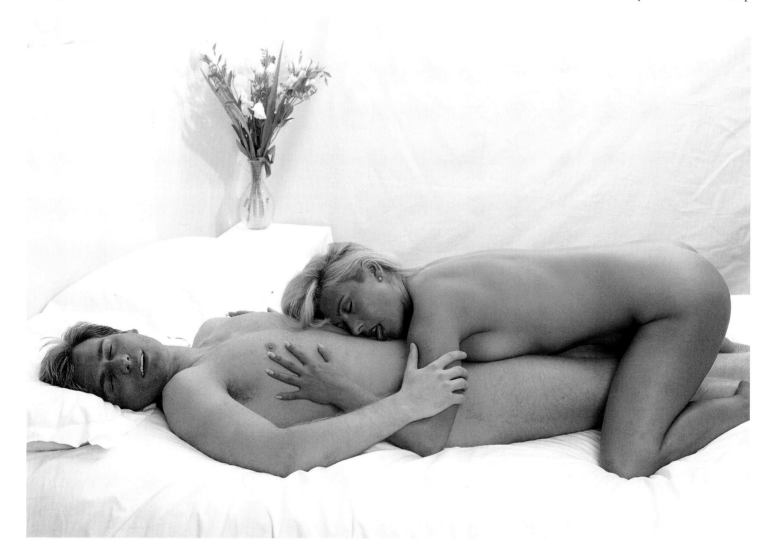

wanting to sleep around (unless they're incredibly immature or stupid – or both). Come the 30s and he's likely to be in a long-term relationship. But the bad news is his desire for sex has dropped a little. In his 40s, a man's output of hormones drops a tiny bit more. Proving that Mother Nature doesn't always get it right, a woman in her 40s is likely to want sex more often!

In his 50s, there's another tiny drop in hormone levels, but 90 per cent of men in this age group are still potent. They can't have one orgasm after another, but their staying power is great. Around 80 per cent of men in their 60s are still potent, wanting and experiencing a good sex life.

It is a sad fact of life that the older one gets, the greater the likelihood that illness will get in the way of the things we enjoy most. A man's sexual performance may be impaired because of ill health and the best tonic a woman can give him is understanding and support – especially armed with the knowledge that at this age an erection is easily lost and not so easily won back. Women, it's down to you to rectify this!

What about the over-70s? In this age group hormone production begins to turn sharply downward in many cases. Sexual capabilities diminish in many men over the age of 70. Again, illness often plays a part in this.

So, while 70 per cent of men are potent at the age of 70, some researchers have found that less than 50 per cent are potent at 75. However, if a man tries to keep himself fit and active, it is certainly possible for him to remain virile until much later than that.

MEN: You may like to know that girls reach puberty at about the same age as boys, but don't

BELOW: Looking for fulfilment can be just as much fun as finding it.

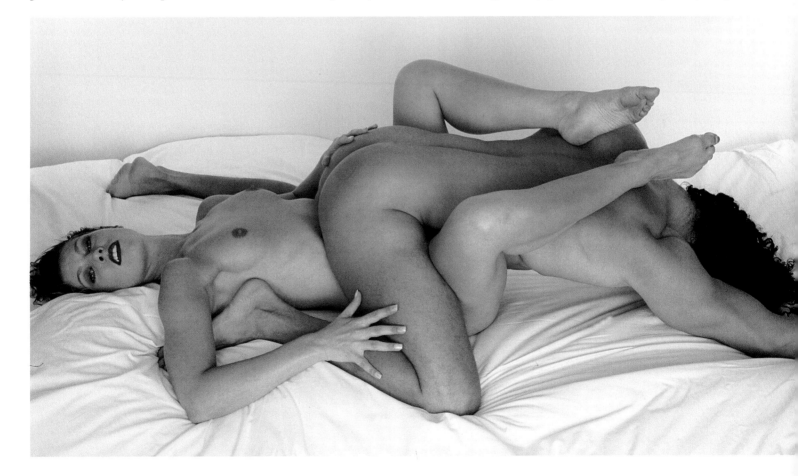

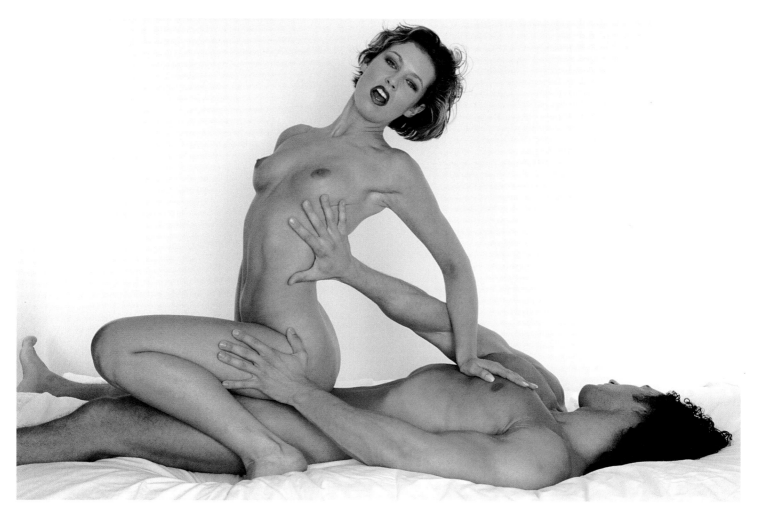

ABOVE: Sex on an angle can be highly stimulating.

usually develop the all-consuming interest in sex that most boys have at this age. Some girls may start masturbating at puberty and this can be very useful in helping them understand how to achieve orgasm.

Most women love sex as much as men by the time they get into their 20s and if lucky enough can have more than one orgasm in a single love-making session. This 'multi-orgasmic' ability increases throughout her 20s and 30s – if she has the right partner.

Women usually start to peak sexually in their 40s, with over 90 per cent regularly enjoying orgasms. A lot of this sexual 'liberation' is down to the fact that an unwanted pregnancy is less likely – though as we know, Mother Nature likes to play tricks – and if you really don't want to get pregnant, take precautions!

Women and the Menopause is a whole new ball game, and warrants far more discussion than we have room for here. Naturally, good old hormones play havoc with your relationship, so men, you *must* be tolerant! Hormones play havoc with the woman's body, too, meaning she will not be as well lubricated for sex as before, or will suffer dreadful sweat attacks or moods making her feel very unlovable. However, recent research has revealed that more women than we think have a trouble-free menopause.

Women can remain very sexually active in their 50s, 60s and 70s, and they are just as capable as men when it comes to taking young lovers. So you see, there may be unexpected variety in your coming years!

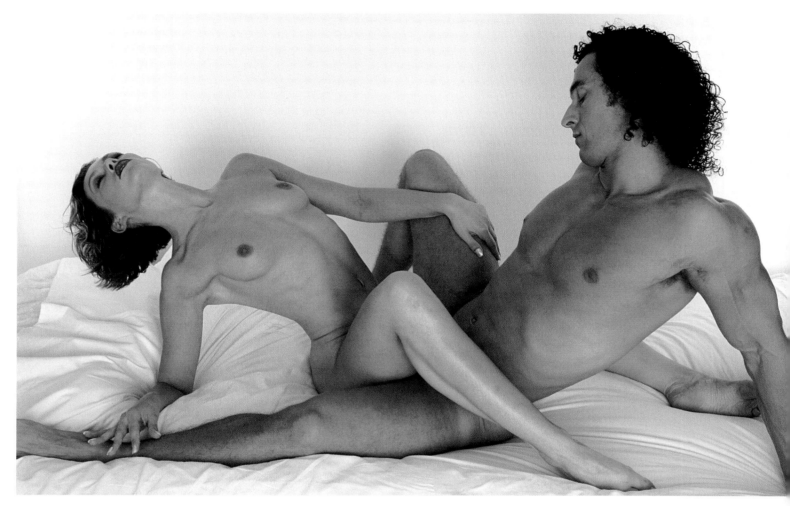

Five Firm Facts about Keeping Fit for Sexual Fulfilment

- Smoking ruins your health and sex life
- So does too much drink
- Too much fatty food slows you down but fibre works fast!
- No one who is overweight has ever been over-sexed
- Exercising mind and body means good stretches of sex

Fulfilment Finale

Would you walk out of a good party without thanking your host or hostess? Or leave a theatre without applauding the show you have just enjoyed? This isn't to suggest you shake hands with your partner or give a round of applause as you both slump on the pillows after your mutually ecstatic love-making, but a nicety is to indulge in 'afterplay'. What greater way to express your love for your partner than to lie in each other's arms, snuggle up against each other and murmur words of contentment. (What isn't appreciated is a 'thank you', which some people have muttered after sex.)

Some believe lighting up a cigarette is a traditional follow-up to sex. There's that old joke, of course: 'Does your partner smoke after sex?' 'I don't know, I've never looked.' You may or may not find that funny. But as was implied earlier in this chapter, smoking is no longer sexy. And aren't lips better used in kissing your partner in appreciative afterplay than propping up a cigarette?

Have a fine sex finale. Have fun sex.

ABOVE: Simultaneous orgasm is the ultimate prize.

6 FUN & GAMES

Don't be shocked! We are about to suggest some of the naughtiest nights (and days) you are ever likely to experience. This is where you let your imagination run riot. Make a sexy video together, pretending that hundreds of eyes are watching you perform… crunch an ice cube in your mouth and have oral sex using your cold tongue and lips on your partner's sexy bits… talk dirty to your partner as you masturbate them. Make a list of 10 things you've never done to each other before – and do them. Enjoy a 'surprise' bout of lovemaking – ensuring she wears a skirt that can easily be lifted up (knickers are optional!) Place mirrors around the bedroom to watch yourselves perform. And these are just a few of the 50 fun games in this chapter. If all of that sounds like a bit of an obstacle course in the ways of love-making, don't despair. Take your time, have lots of fun and fantasy, and hopefully you'll soon be going around with big smiles on your faces!

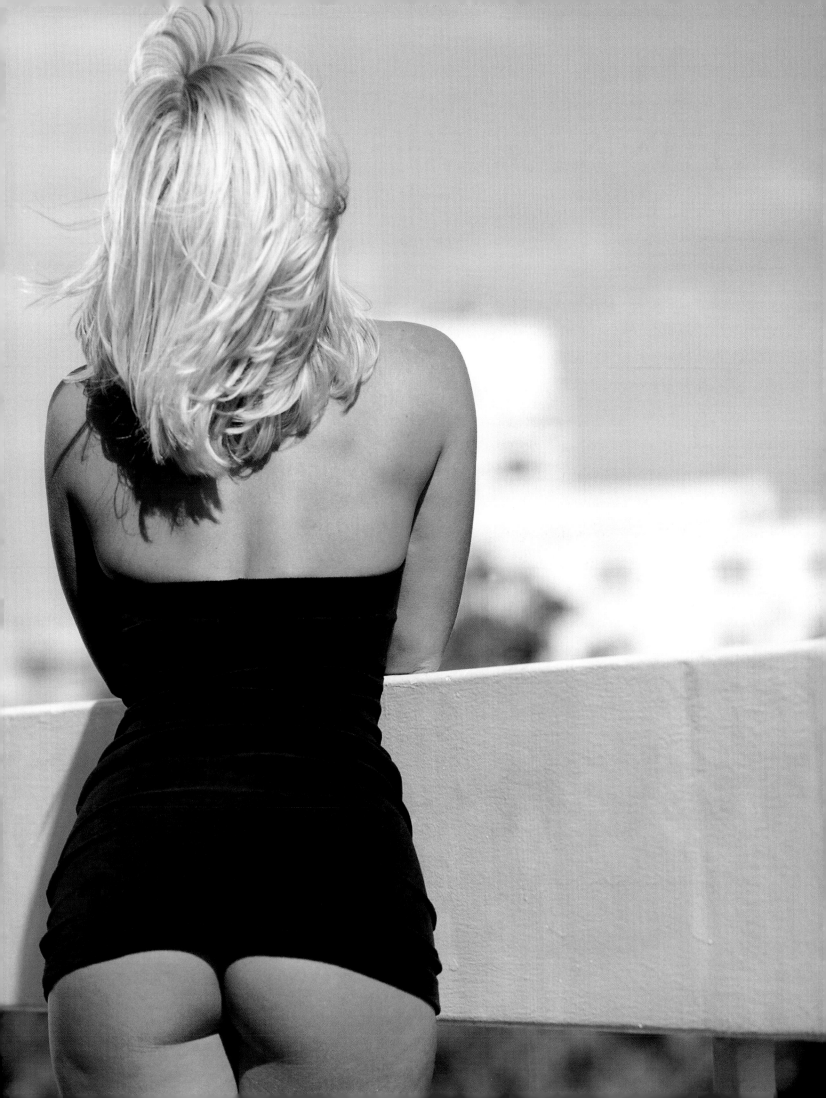

There is a reason why this book is called *Fun Sex* – because it's aimed at bringing love, laughter, fun and games back into your sex life. Quite a tall order, you may agree.

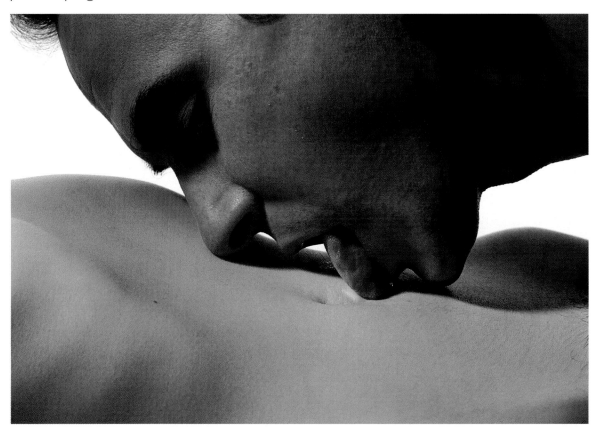

RIGHT: Be inventive and let your imagination run riot.

Best if you and your partner have been reading these pages together, you should know there are other positions other than the missionary and that love-making isn't only to be savoured at the weekend. Hopefully you are well on the way to going around with big smiles on your faces.

There's so much to be had from lots of fun, fantasies and a bit of devilment when you try something new on the sex front. Though, as should always be stressed, anything you do has to be fun for both of you.

This chapter is simple. It's where you can really let your imagination run riot. It's 50 quick ways to have more fun in the bedroom – or preferably somewhere other than the bedroom. So read on, and even if you only have a go at half of them, your sex life will be half as good again!

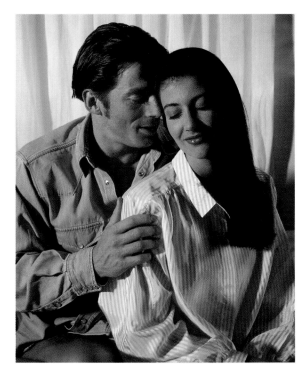

RIGHT: Prepare yourself for an intense experience!

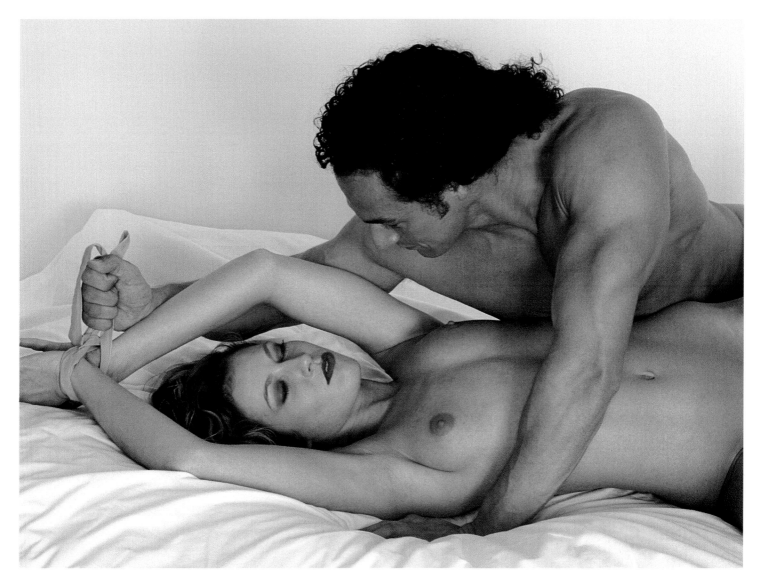

1. Pin her arms above her head when you make love tonight. She gets to tie yours up when it's her turn.

2. Talk dirty to your partner as you masturbate them, or say you will 'punish' them if they orgasm too quickly.

3. Use spray cream to smother your partner's sexiest bits then lick it off in exactly the time they set you. A forfeit if you fail to please.

4. Make the room as dark as possible and get your partner to lie down (totally naked and vulnerable, of course). Leave them there, only to return after a few deliciously teasing minutes. Then in total silence, ravish your partner in as many ways as you can.

5. This one is *not* to be taken too seriously – we don't want undue stress here! Give your partner a set time to bring you to orgasm. If they fail, think of a sexual forfeit they have to perform. If they succeed, they choose exactly what you have to do to them.

6. Take it in turns to undress each other. To slow the game down, just undo one button or zip. To speed it up, remove whole items of clothing. Or you might like to mix and match!

7. Lie naked beside each other and choose who starts the 'touching game'. Beginning at the feet, caress and fondle as sensually as you can. The recipient gives marks out of ten for how much your fondling of various parts of their body turns them on.

LEFT: Pin your partner's arms up above her head while you have sex.

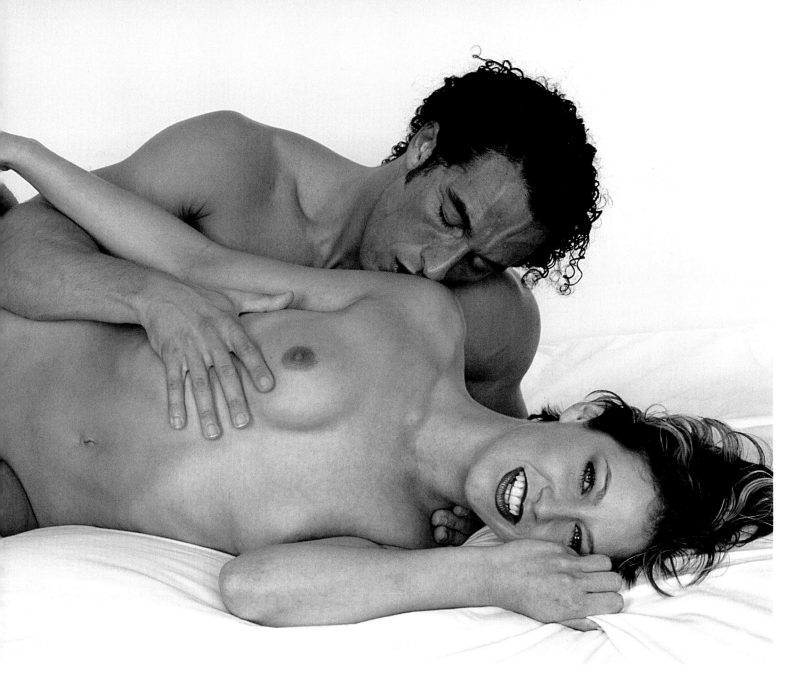

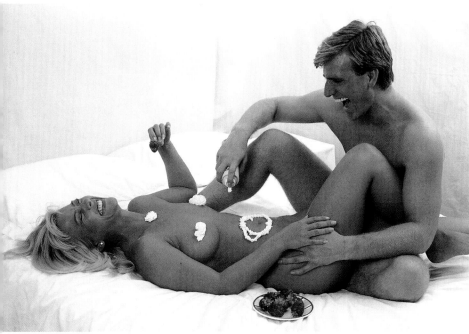

8. Massage your partner's body in sensual, slow strokes, gently teasing around the genital area but *not* actually touching it. Then restrain your partner's arms and legs with silken ropes and perform oral sex.

9. Enjoy a 'surprise' bout of love-making. Ensure she wears a skirt that can easily be lifted up. Knickers are optional. Kiss and cuddle her from behind, all the while telling her what you are going to do. Then make her face a wall with her hands pressed against it. Lift up her dress or skirt and enter her. (It's difficult to have the same element of surprise with the man taking the passive role, but you can always fondle him when he's pre-occupied and see where it leads.)

10. Make a sexy video together, pretending that hundreds of eyes are watching you perform. But the deal is that the finished film is for your eyes only, so this particular bit of sex fun is only for the totally trustworthy.

11. Enjoy your own brand of oral sex with her 'kissing' your mouth with her vagina and you kissing hers with your penis. The recipient is not allowed to move.

12. Set yourselves the challenge of making love over or on every piece of furniture in the house.

13. Be unfaithful – with your partner! Arrange to meet at a hotel and pretend you are having an extra-marital affair. Arrive separately, have a drink or dinner together, then retire to the bedroom. One partner might like to call the other at work at out of the blue and set the time and venue. Some couples play this game at home – even going as far as to suddenly say, 'Hurry, my husband's coming.'

14. Get rid of the television for a week. You'll be surprised at how much earlier you want to go to bed. As part of an experiment, one small town in America gave up watching television for a month. The number of times couples had sex increased dramatically.

15. Write down on pieces of paper various weird and wonderful ways of making love. Screw the notes into balls, mix them all up, then pick out as many as you like. The only rule of this game is that you have to do everything you have picked out. You may want to limit it to one or two ways, or take it in turns, letting your partner write all the directions on alternate nights. There's delicious anticipation in hearing what you are going to do.

16. One of you hides in part of the house (the more unusual the better) and the other looks for them. Then you make love.

17. Your favourite food doesn't always have to be served on a plate! Why not ask your partner to present it to you on their own naked body. You don't need cutlery, of course – just use your lips and tongue.

18. Play Sexy Scrabble in which *only* suggestive words can be made. The naughtier the better – especially if you say, 'This is what I'm thinking about right now' as you place the letters on the board.

19. Plan a film show at home. Make sure you set the scene to make both of you feel as relaxed as possible, including wearing comfortable, easily-removed clothes. Then run through a sexy video or two, adding your own commentary as you go.

20. Buy tickets to the cinema but sit in separate seats, making sure you know where each other is. After a while, one of you moves in the seat next to the other and pretends to be a 'groper', fondling their partner and going as far as possible (without causing offence to those around you or breaking the law!).

21. Crunch an ice cube in your mouth then have oral sex using your cold tongue and lips on your partner's sensitive sexy bits.

22. Wake up, set an exact time that day you are going to have sex and do it. (Be cautious over where you might be at the time.)

OPPOSITE ABOVE: *Fun, fantasies and a bit of devilishness are the keys when trying something new on the sex front.*

OPPOSITE BELOW: *Whip yourself up into a frenzy by eating your favourite food off your partner's naked body.*

BELOW: *Pretend you are having an illicit affair – with your partner. Meet up in your bedroom or even a hotel!*

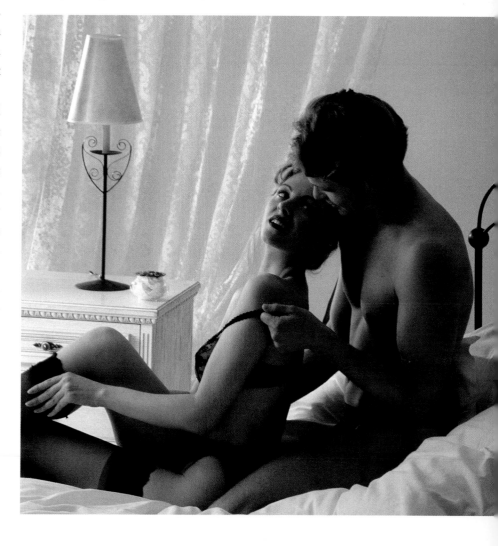

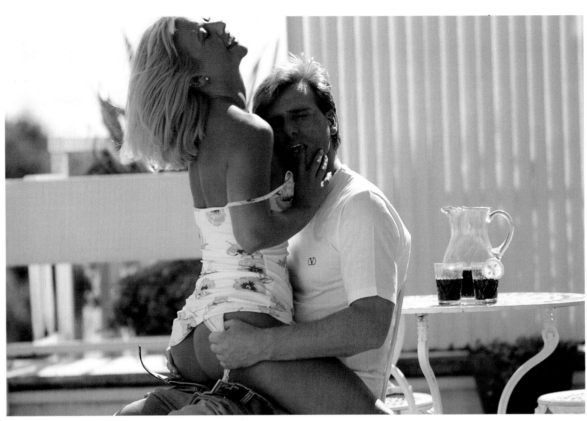

RIGHT: Anyone watching? Pretend you are having a "quickie" in a public place.

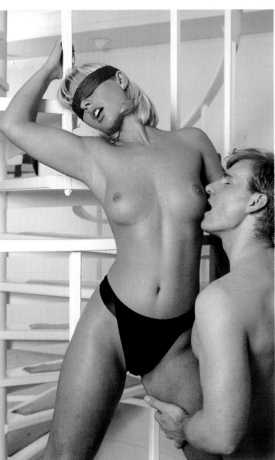

ABOVE: Use a blindfold to close off one sense and heighten the others.

23. Give each other an exotic foot massage. Oil your feet and use them to massage your partner's penis or vagina.

24. Place mirrors around the bedroom to watch yourselves perform. You might like to pretend they are two-way mirrors and you are being observed.

25. Make a telephone call while your partner is arousing you and see how long you can carry on a conversation without responding.

26. Make it a challenge to work your way through the *Karma Sutra*. A lot of it looks impossible, but improvisation can be a lot more fun!

27. Play the game 'Twister' and have sex in the most ludicrous position you end up in.

28. Have '69' sex and whoever makes their partner orgasm first is in charge of that session's sex play.

29. One night let him play the 'Prostitute and Client' game, so long as you get to play the 'Paid Stud and Client' game.

30. Pretend you are having an illicit 'quickie' and both keep your pants on during sex.

31. Closing off one sense heightens the others, so why not use a blindfold, headphones or even a gag (which needs a lot of trust) to stimulate your sense of anticipation?

32. Play caller and sex line operator. And it doesn't have to be the man that telephones to hear sex talk – swap roles for added excitement.

33. Each make a list of ten things you have never done to each other before – and do them.

34. Agree on a secret sign that leads you to have a 'quickie' in a quiet place at a party.

35. One of you is the virgin for the night and the other is the sex education teacher!

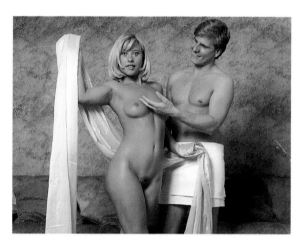

36. Take it in turns to show each other how you can give yourself an orgasm.

37. Pretend your naked body is on exhibition. Strike a pose. Your partner is the curious visitor who tweaks and touches. (You can't move – you're an exhibit!)

38. Imagine you're the prize in a raffle and your partner is the winner who can do anything he likes with you.

39. You can't beat the old favourites – so how about a game of doctors and nurses?

40. Both write down a numbered list of six sexy people you admire. Don't show each other your lists, but get your partner to call out a number, blindfold them, and 'give' them their fantasy partner.

41. Lie down, close your eyes and imagine your partner is two people taking it in turns to do different things to you.

42. Men, pretend you're a male stripper who's scored with a member of the audience; women, pretend you're a lap-dancer and things have gone too far.

LEFT: Stay as still as a statue and let your partner touch you wherever they fancy.

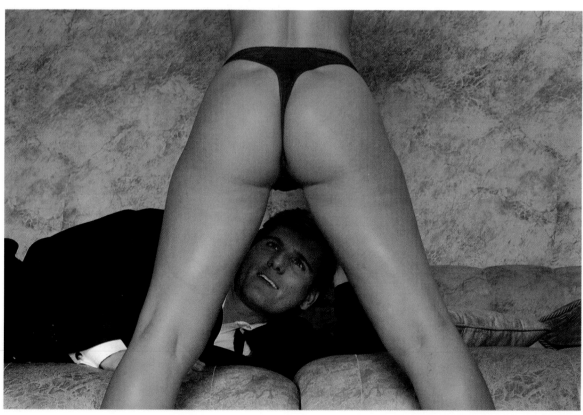

LEFT: Lap dancing gone too far.

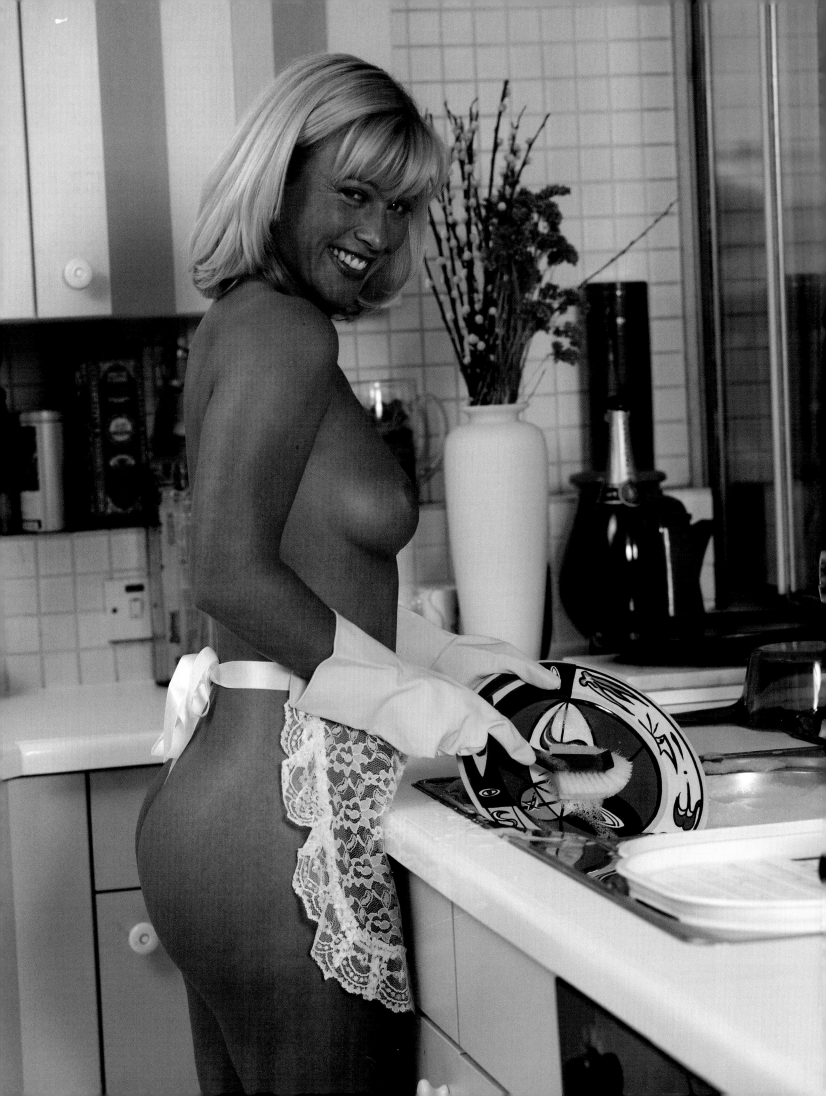

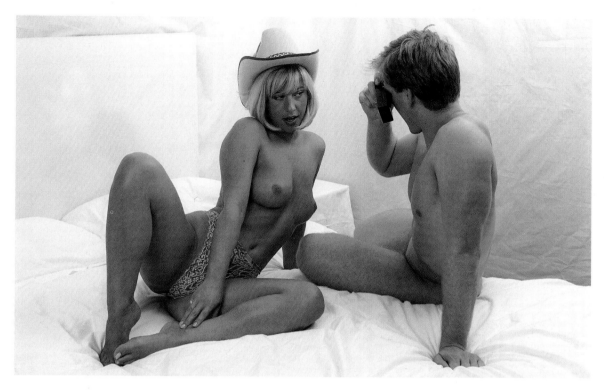

43. Dress in each other's clothing and swap roles (pretending to be your partner) or simply enjoy the sexy strangeness of it all. (This is one occasion when size really does matter!)

44. Pose for naughty pictures in the fantasy that they are going to be published in a magazine. (Safe if only the two of you are involved, but safer fun with no film in the camera while you are posing.)

45. Only try this one in a deserted place: Tie your partner to a tree, 'hide' for a few moments, then return as if a stranger coming upon a defenceless 'victim' in the wood. What you do next is down to you, but something of a sexy nature is recommended.

46. Pretend you are a sex slave that your 'master' or 'mistress' keeps for the amusement and at the mercy of their friends.

47. With your partner tied and blindfolded, blow gently across every part of their naked body.

48. Get your partner to perform normal tasks but in the nude, e.g. washing up, vacuuming or washing the car (preferably in the garage!).

49. Massage him with your breasts; massage her with your penis.

50. Have a pillow fight. It will make you feel like kids again, but should lead to adult fun.

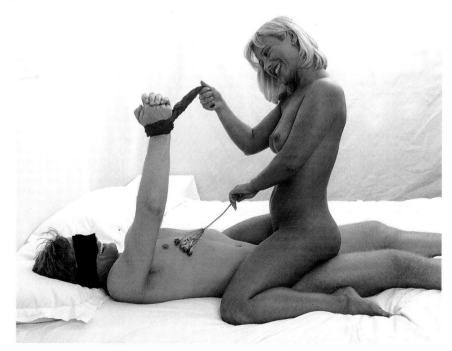

INDEX